Hair to Dye For

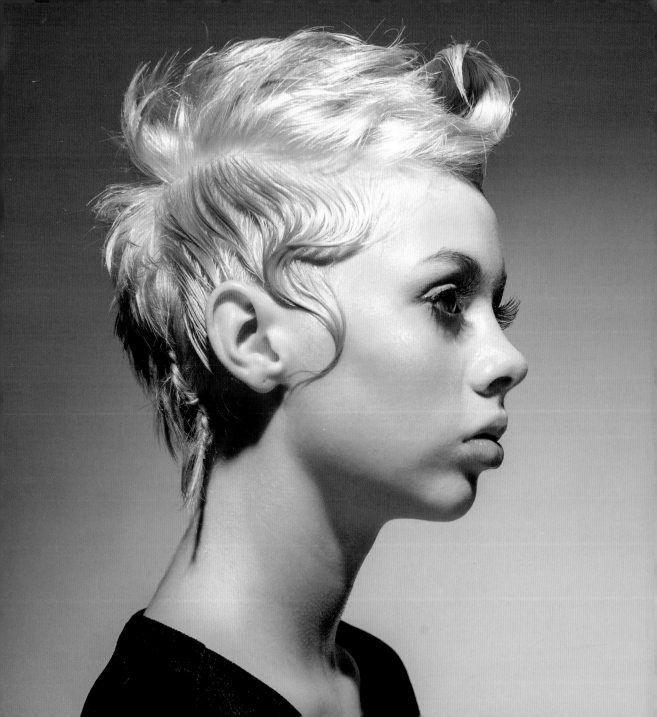

ASH FORTIS XO HAIR LAB

Hair to Dye For

Photography by
Glenn Fajota

weldonowen

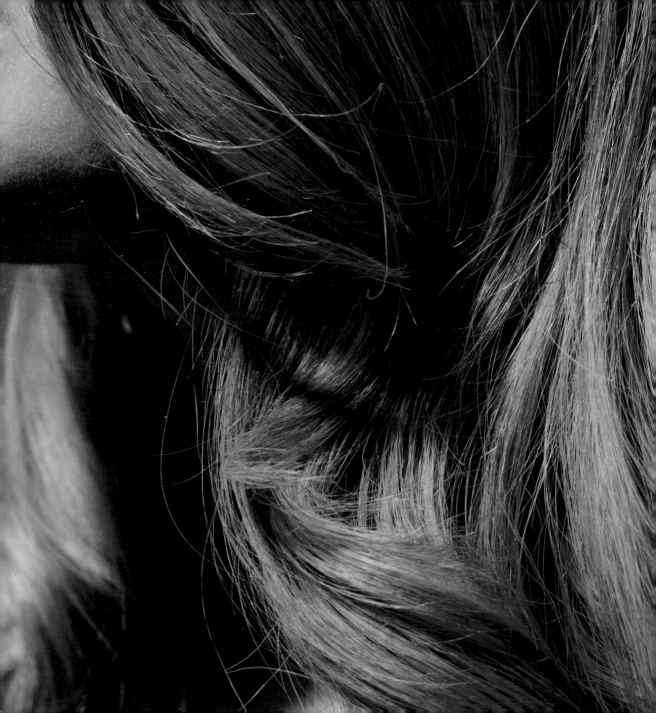

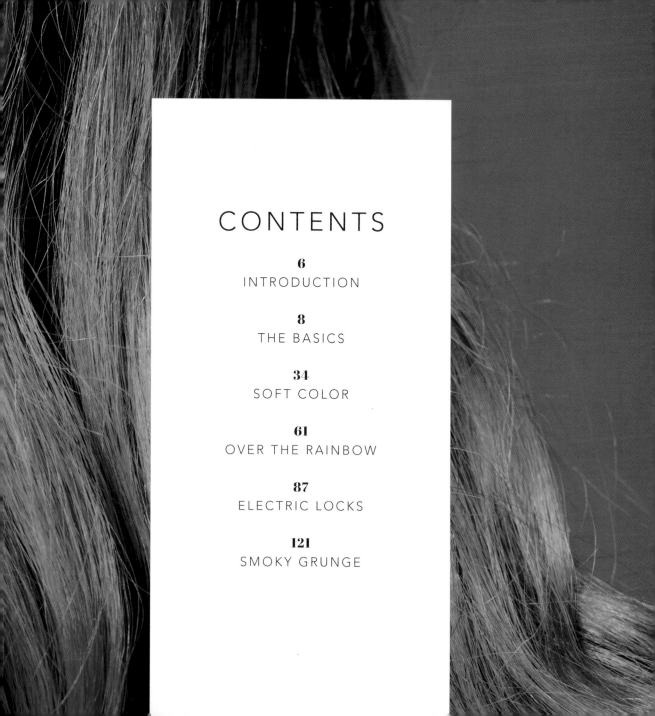

CONTENTS

A Passion for Transformation

I'VE ALWAYS LOVED COLOR AND STYLE, AND EVEN AS A LITTLE KID I WAS EXPERIMENTING—WITH MY OWN HAIR, AS WELL AS ON FRIENDS, FAMILY, AND ANYONE ELSE WILLING TO TRUST AN UNLICENSED 12-YEAR-OLD "STYLIST." OUT OF THOSE EXPERIMENTS (SOME MORE SUCCESSFUL THAN OTHERS!) CAME MY FANSTATIC CAREER AS A STYLIST AND EDUCATOR. I'VE ALWAYS LOVED HELPING PEOPLE FIND THE RIGHT LOOK, AND IN THIS BOOK, I SHARE SOME OF MY FAVORITE CREATIVE COLOR EFFECTS, WITH STEP-BY-STEP INSTRUCTIONS. WHETHER YOU'RE A DIY BEGINNER OR A SEASONED STYLIST, THIS BOOK HAS THE INFORMATION AND INSPIRATION YOU NEED TO FIND THE PERFECT LOOK.

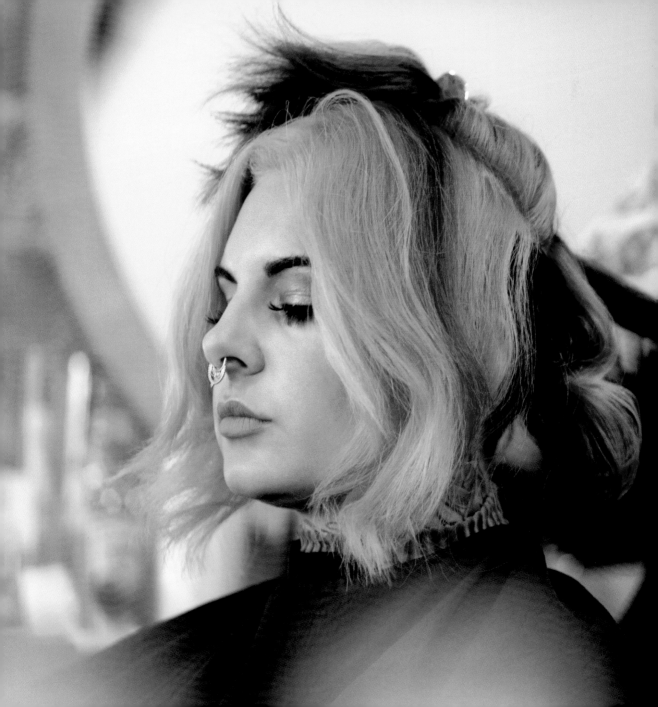

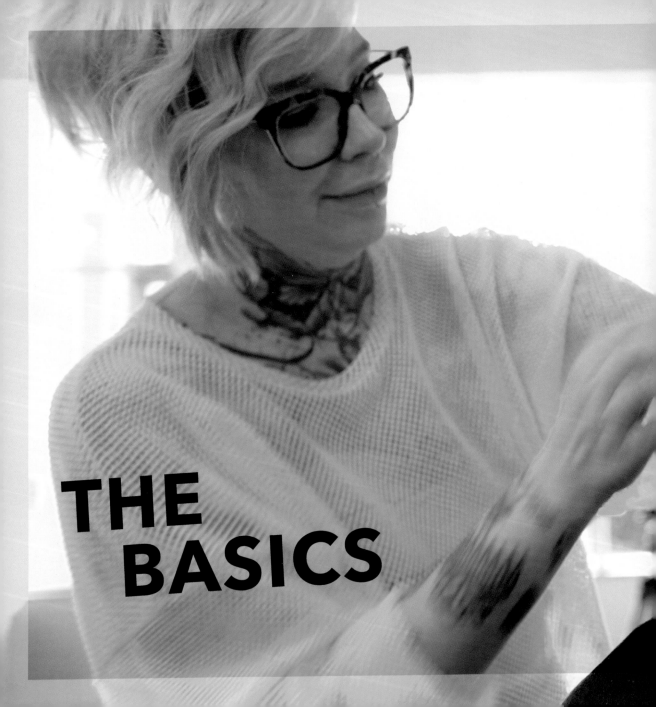

THE
BASICS

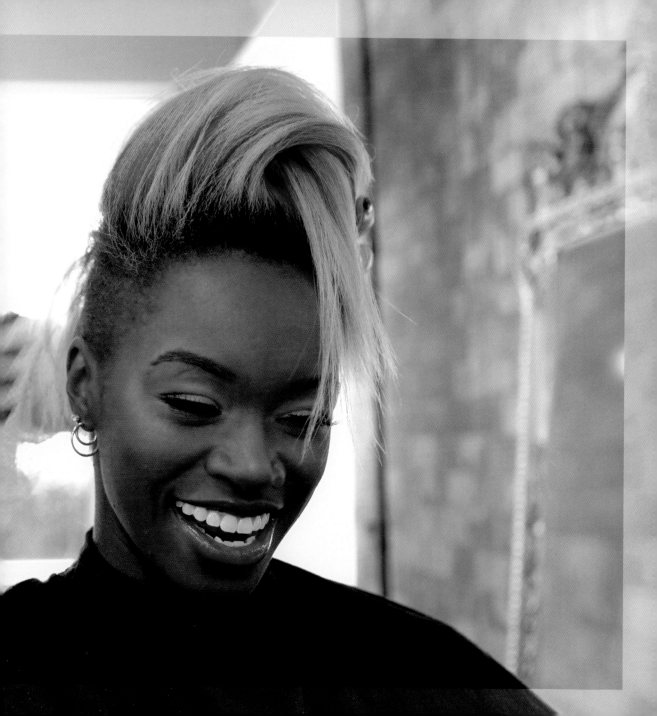

Get Started

IN THE CHAPTER THAT FOLLOWS, WE'RE GOING TO GO OVER ALL THE THINGS YOU'LL NEED TO KNOW BEFORE YOU BEGIN, FROM FIGURING OUT YOUR HAIR'S TEXTURE AND COLOR TO CHOOSING THE RIGHT PRODUCTS, BEING SURE YOU HAVE ALL THE TOOLS YOU NEED, AND UNDERSTANDING SOME BASIC TERMINOLOGY. IN ADDITION, WE'LL GO OVER SOME OFTEN-MISUNDERSTOOD INS AND OUTS OF COLOR THEORY, TO BE SURE YOU GET THE RESULTS YOU WERE EXPECTING. WE'LL MAKE SURE YOU KNOW HOW TO TAKE CARE OF YOUR FABULOUS NEW COLOR AND ENSURE IT LASTS AS LONG AS POSSIBLE—UNTIL YOU'RE READY TO TRY SOMETHING NEW AND EQUALLY AWESOME!

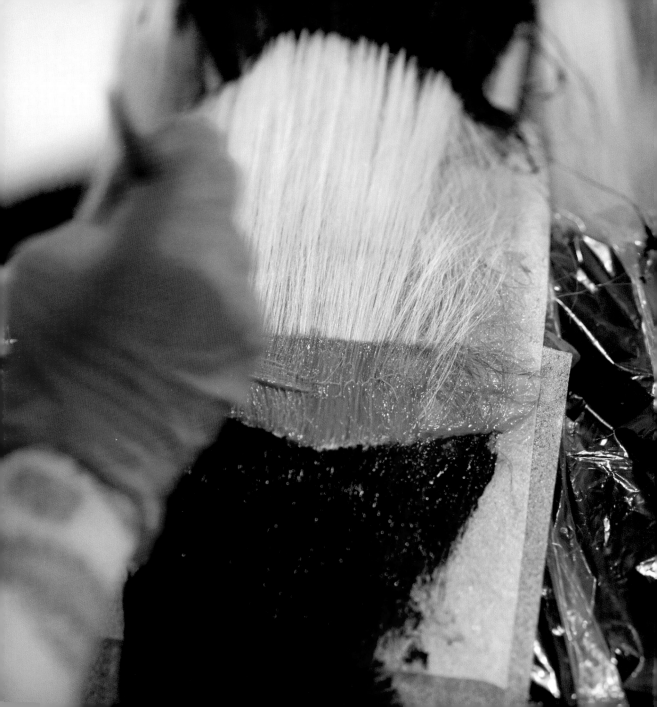

KNOW YOUR HAIR

Before you even get to thinking about color, you'll want to start with the big picture. We talk about your hair as the canvas, the starting point for creating your work of art.

TYPE AND TEXTURE The two factors here are how straight or curly the individual hairs are, and how thick. Hair type is described as 1 (straight), 2 (wavy), 3 (curly), or 4 (kinky). Within those categories, "a" is the finest hair texture, "b" is medium, and "c" is the coarsest. Knowing your hair type and texture helps you understand how your hair will take color, and what additional steps you might need to take. For example, someone with very fine, straight 1 hair presents a different set of advantages and challenges than someone with very thick, tightly kinked 4c hair.

The fine, light 1a hair is very easy to apply color to, with no twists and turns to navigate. But it's also likely to be very slippery, and hard to section or to pin up out of the way while working.

Hair at the other end of the scale is very easy to section and to secure with clips—in fact, if the hair is short and thick enough, you might not even need to pin it, as it stay in place beautifully. However, this hair is also likely to resist lightening and to be difficult to saturate with color. In the tutorials throughout this book, we note interesting challenges we faced with each model, which can help you get a sense of what to expect.

DENSITY This is what's meant by "thick" or "thin" hair, although many people confuse this with the size of the individual strands. But any hair type can be thicker or thinner. To determine your hair's density, take a front section of your hair and pull it to the side. If you can visibly see sections of your scalp underneath or through the hair, then your hair is thin. If you barely see your scalp at all, your hair is thick. If it's somewhere in-between, then your hair has a medium density. The denser your hair, the more color you'll need for full coverage.

POROSITY This refers to how easily your hair absorbs moisture. Low porosity hair tends to dry quickly and may not absorb product well. High porosity hair can take forever to dry, but absorbs product easily. Uneven porosity hair, often the result of overprocessing, may take color unevenly. To determine your hair's porosity, there are two simple tests you can do. For the Float Test, just take a couple of strands of your hair, drop them into a bowl of water, and let them sit for a few minutes. If the hair floats, you have low porosity. If it sinks, you have high porosity. An even simpler test is the Slip'n'Slide Test. Just slide your fingers up one hair toward your scalp. If you feel little bumps along the way, this means that your cuticle is lifted and that you have high porosity. If your fingers slip smoothly, then you have low porosity hair.

TYPE 1: STRAIGHT HAIR
Fine to Coarse, Curl Resistant

1A **1B** **1C**

TYPE 2: WAVY HAIR
Fine to Thin to Coarse and Frizzy

2A **2B** **2C**

TYPE 3: CURLY HAIR
Loose Curly to Corkscrew Curly

3A **3B** **3C**

TYPE 4: KINKY HAIR
Tightly Coiled to Z-angled Coils

4A **4B** **4C**

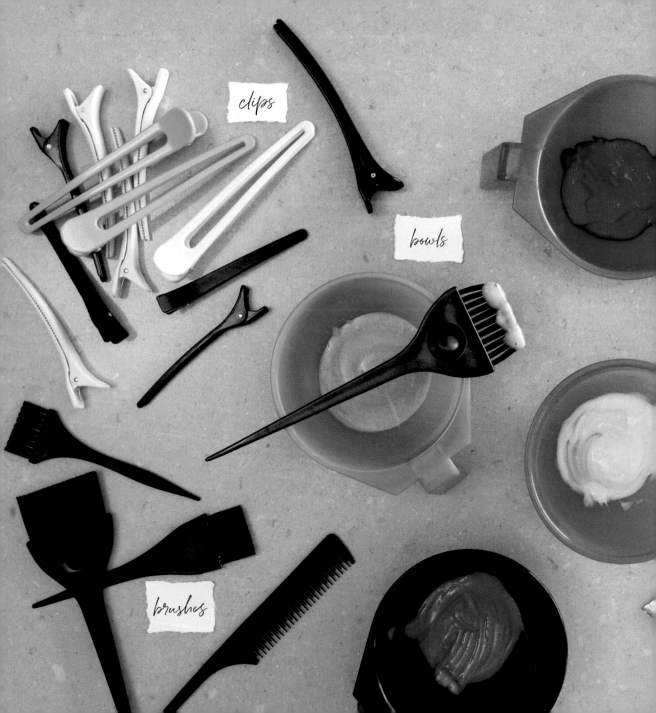

clips

bowls

brushes

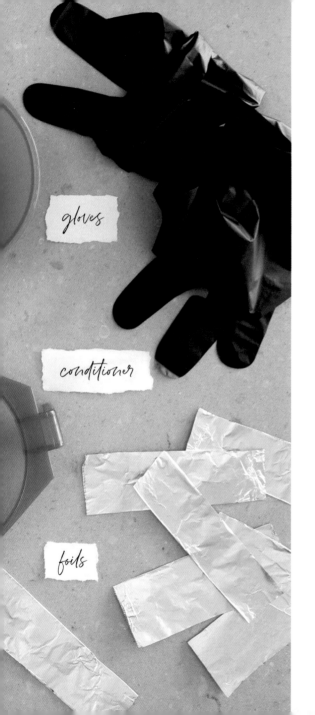

gloves

conditioner

foils

TOOLS OF THE TRADE

You can spend many hours and dollars at your local beauty store, but you don't really need that much. Here are the basics.

CAPE Protect your clothing with a hair stylist's cape or an old towel you don't mind staining.

CLIPS Use clips to keep hair out of the way while you're working; choose plastic over metal, as metal clips can rust and discolor your hair.

CONDITIONER Mix any white conditioner with a small amount of dye to create a pastel version, or mix it with violet dye to make homemade toner.

GLOVES Protect your hands at all times—even semipermanent color can stain skin.

BRUSH There is no substitute for proper coloring brushes. The pointy ends are great for sectioning, while the bristles apply dye with precision.

MIXING BOWLS You can mix your color up in any glass or plastic bowl that doesn't stain, but the purpose-made bowls make application easy.

COMB A rat-tail comb helps with sectioning, and you'll often want to comb through the applied dye.

FOILS To keep sections separate, use store-bought foils or cut your own from tinfoil.

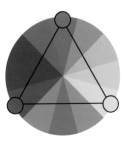

Primary

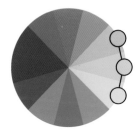

Analogous

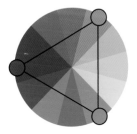

Secondary

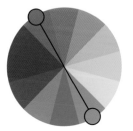

Complementary

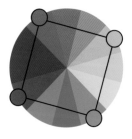

Square

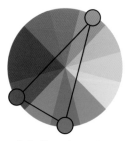

Split Complementary

COLOR THEORY

The color wheel might not seem relevant to hair and beauty, but in fact a little color theory can make a massive difference in your success with your creative looks. As you may remember from grammar school, there are three **primary colors**: red, yellow, and blue. Most of the other colors in the rainbow can be made by mixing those three in the right proportions, the simplest mixes being the **secondary colors**.

When you use semipermanent colors, the end result will be a mix of you base color and the dye. That's why even the brightest color applied over brown hair will tend to be dull and muddy. If your hair has strong yellow tones and you try to dye it sky blue, your end result will actually be green (yellow + blue = green). That's why we recommend lightening your hair to a neutral tone before applying dye, to get the truest tone.

The theory of **complementary colors** is particularly helpful. This states that opposite colors neutralize each other. That's why a violet toner will almost magically remove overly yellow tones from lightened hair. **Analogous colors** are the closest cousins on the wheel, so look to these groupings for a subtle multicolor effect. For high-contrast combinations, look to **split complementary** schemes, with one dominant color and two complements, or the **square** range, which mixes four strong opposites for a dynamic effect.

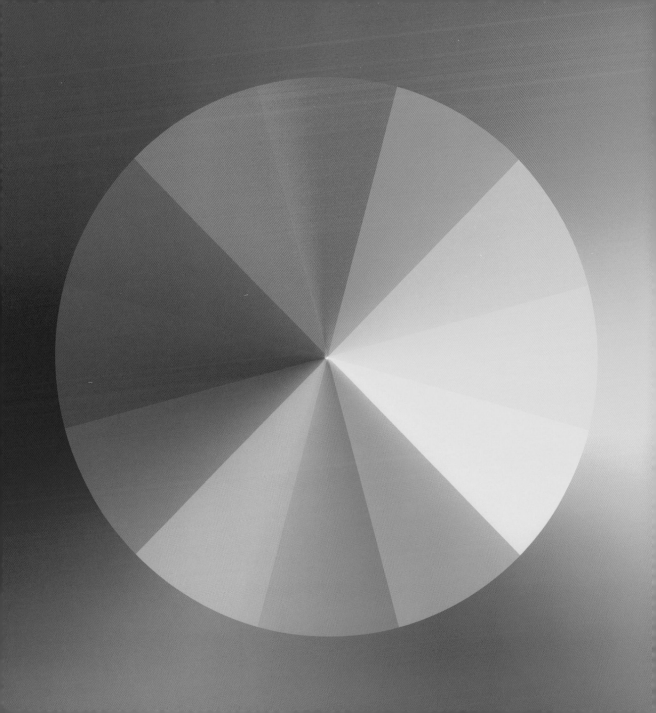

HAIR COLOR LEVELS

When we talk about natural or chemically lightened hair, we need to be speaking the same language. After all, one person's "medium reddish brown" might be another's "dark strawberry blonde." Hair professionals have solved this problem with the system shown here, a universal numbering code that goes from darkest black (1) to lightest blonde (10). Once we start getting into bleached hair, we may go as high as 12 or 13 for whitest platinum.

To figure out which level you are, take a section of your hair and hold it up away from the rest of the hair to isolate it and get some light on it. The hair around your face tends to be the lightest, so choose a piece from farther back, near the crown. Compare that strand to this chart—if you're not sure, call in a friend to help you figure it out, or ask a professional stylist for their input next time you visit a salon.

The other really useful thing to know here is the hair's dominant underlying pigment, which will be revealed in the lightening process. You'll generally have to keep hair's underlying pigment in mind when you are lightening two shades or more from the natural hair color. Sometimes you can use this to good effect—if you've got Level 4 dark brown hair and want a crazy vibrant orange, for example, you'll be able to build on the natural pigments. If your end goal is a cool icy pastel green, you'll want to plan on a lot more neutralizing.

NATURAL HAIR COLOR LEVELS

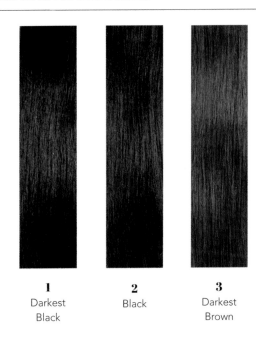

1
Darkest
Black

2
Black

3
Darkest
Brown

UNDERLYING EXPOSED PIGMENT

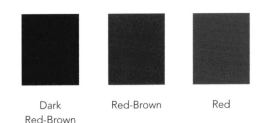

Dark
Red-Brown

Red-Brown

Red

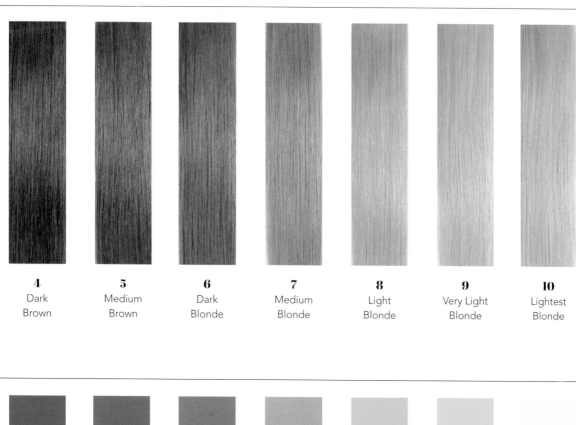

| **4**
Dark
Brown | **5**
Medium
Brown | **6**
Dark
Blonde | **7**
Medium
Blonde | **8**
Light
Blonde | **9**
Very Light
Blonde | **10**
Lightest
Blonde |

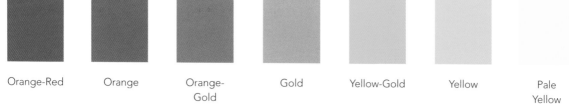

| Orange-Red | Orange | Orange-
Gold | Gold | Yellow-Gold | Yellow | Pale
Yellow |

COLOR IN ACTION

Okay, we've talked about hair color levels and pigments, and we've taken a spin around the color wheel. How will all of this theory play out in real life? Glad you asked! My signature color line, Pulp Riot, has created this handy chart to show how different colors will look when applied to the hair levels we recommend will work best with them (which vary, as the darker colors will work on a wider range of tones; the lighter colors need a fairly light canvas to start with). These swatches show my Pulp Riot colors in action, but you can extrapolate from them to imagine how semipermanent colors from any maker will work for you.

For example, let's say you have Level 6 brown hair and love the look of Cupid, a hot pink color. If you don't lighten your natural hair color before applying Cupid, the result will be a rich but fairly subtle magenta. On Level 10 hair, the same pigment will be a very striking, almost neon pink. Both look great, and with this chart, you'll be able to predict which you'll get (and how might you need to lighten for the more vibrant effect.)

Some colors, like Seaglass (a vibrant green) and Lilac are only recommended for the lightest hair levels, as their pale tones need a lighter canvas to really shine. Armed with this information, you should be able to color mix and match like a pro.

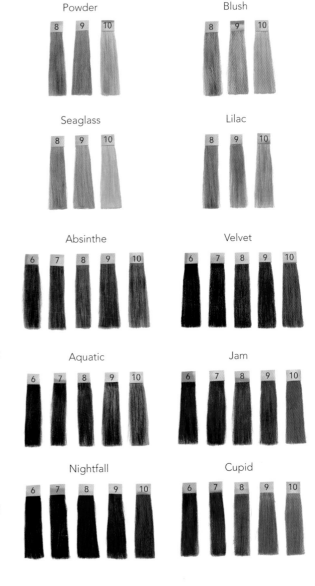

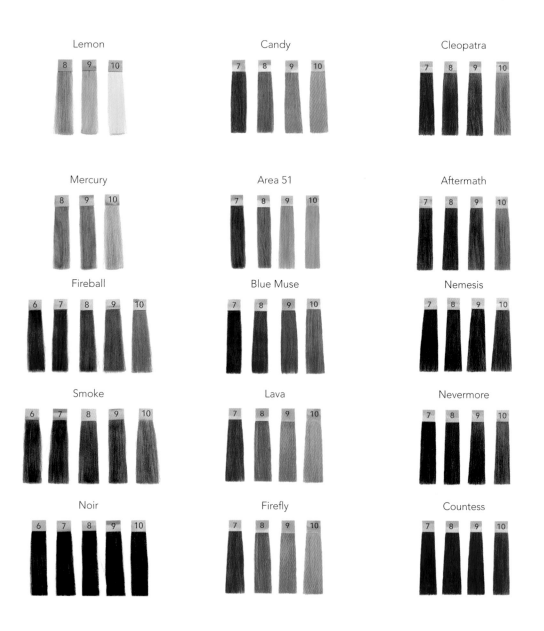

Lemon

| 8 | 9 | 10 |

Candy

| 7 | 8 | 9 | 10 |

Cleopatra

| 7 | 8 | 9 | 10 |

Mercury

| 8 | 9 | 10 |

Area 51

| 7 | 8 | 9 | 10 |

Aftermath

| 7 | 8 | 9 | 10 |

Fireball

| 6 | 7 | 8 | 9 | 10 |

Blue Muse

| 7 | 8 | 9 | 10 |

Nemesis

| 7 | 8 | 9 | 10 |

Smoke

| 6 | 7 | 8 | 9 | 10 |

Lava

| 7 | 8 | 9 | 10 |

Nevermore

| 7 | 8 | 9 | 10 |

Noir

| 6 | 7 | 8 | 9 | 10 |

Firefly

| 7 | 8 | 9 | 10 |

Countess

| 7 | 8 | 9 | 10 |

PICKING YOUR PAINT

Most of the effects in this book are achieved using semipermanent colors applied to prelightened hair, although a few of the looks rely on demi colors. While of course I use Pulp Riot, the color line I helped create, you can use any high-quality semipermanent brand: Manic Panic, Crazy Color, Arctic Fox, Ion, and Adore are just some of the brands you can find in beauty stores or online. Read reviews, look at available colors, and make your choice accordingly. It's okay to mix different brands together, although some have very different consistencies (for example, Ion is notoriously thick and intense, while Adore is much more liquid), so take this into account if you are mixing brands.

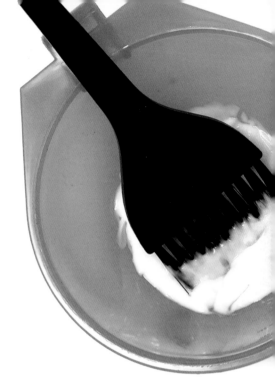

LIGHTENING Most of the effects in this book are designed to pop on prelightened hair. Some start with an ombre, sombre, or balayage (see page 26), others with the canvas lightened overall. Lifting color, whether that's removing an existing dye job or lightening your natural color, can be tricky, and doing it wrong can damage your hair. If you don't have experience working with bleach, please have a professional take care of this step for you—and then you can play with color at home to your heart's content!

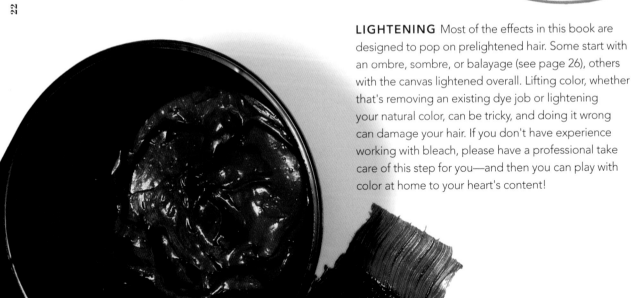

SEMIPERMANENT COLOR

This conditioner-based color is the formulation most commonly used to achieve fun creative colors, from soft pastels to wild neon tones. Semipermanent dyes do not lift or change your original hair color. Instead, they coat the hair shaft in a colorful, conditioning dye. If you care for your color carefully it can last for a couple of months, although for many people it will largely wash out over 12 to 14 shampoos.

DEMIPERMANENT COLOR

As you might guess from its name, demipermanent color exists on a spectrum between semipermanent colors (described above) and permanent colors, which are the more traditional peroxide-based colors you see on drugstore shelves. Demis, as they're known, use a low-intensity peroxide (often as low as a 6 or 10 volume) to develop the color, which means it does lift your base color very slightly. Demis will penetrate the hair shaft rather than coating it, which mean they are longer lasting. Some effects use both demi and semipermanent colors for different stages, but you shouldn't mix the dyes together as they work differently.

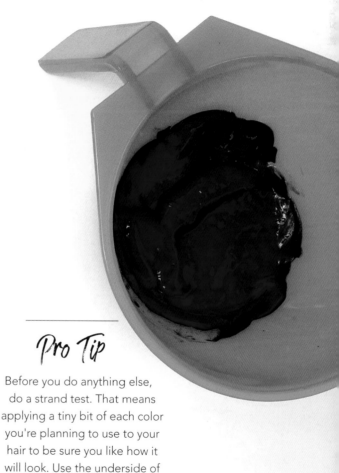

Pro Tip

Before you do anything else, do a strand test. That means applying a tiny bit of each color you're planning to use to your hair to be sure you like how it will look. Use the underside of a pre-lightened strand so that any less-than-awesome results are out of view.

READ A HEADSHEET

Headsheets are one of those wonderful tools that stylists rely on (for cut, color, and more) but that are little known outside the professional world. Essentially, a headsheet is a sketch that gives you guidance on how and where to apply the dye to achieve a specific effect. Throughout this book, we've provided headsheets for many of the looks, to help guide your hand. Be aware that this is much more of an art than a science. You may want to apply slightly different colors, and that's fine! In addition, different hair types (see page 12) will dictate different sectioning. We'll often show a single section in the headsheet, but a person with very dense, fine hair might require multiple sections in that area for full coverage. And, of course, longer or shorter hair will require some adjustments.

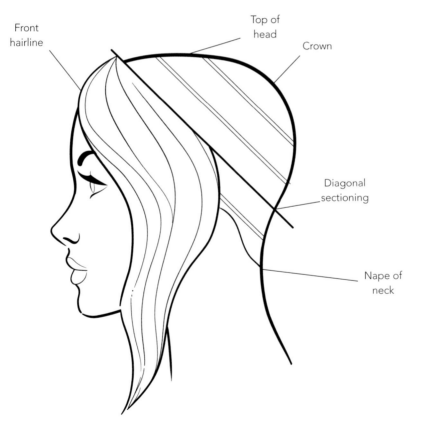

Front hairline

Top of head

Crown

Diagonal sectioning

Nape of neck

In addition to showing you which colors are applied where, the headsheet shows you how to section the hair for coloring. In general, the diagram will only show one full lock of hair if every lock is supposed to get the same treatment. When you see more locks drawn, that's a cue that different sections will be getting different dye patterns or colors.

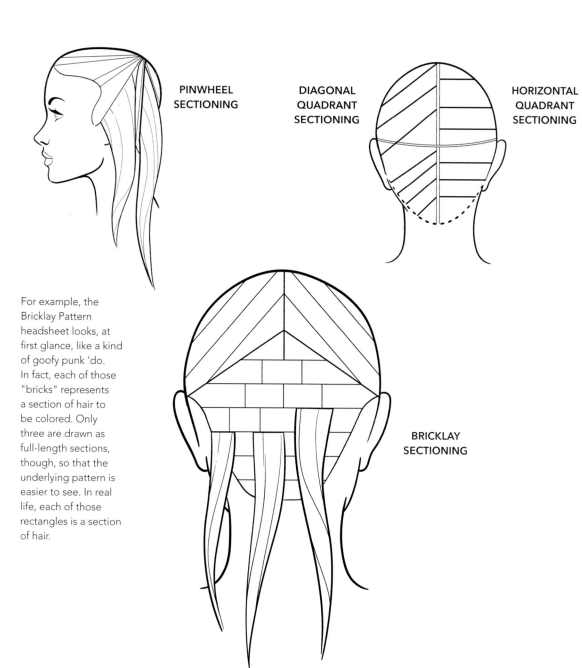

PINWHEEL
SECTIONING

DIAGONAL
QUADRANT
SECTIONING

HORIZONTAL
QUADRANT
SECTIONING

For example, the
Bricklay Pattern
headsheet looks, at
first glance, like a kind
of goofy punk 'do.
In fact, each of those
"bricks" represents
a section of hair to
be colored. Only
three are drawn as
full-length sections,
though, so that the
underlying pattern is
easier to see. In real
life, each of those
rectangles is a section
of hair.

BRICKLAY
SECTIONING

OMBRE, SOMBRE & BALAYAGE

Multilevel lightening techniques are very popular as a way to bring dimensionality and interest to natural hair tones, even if no additional color is being added to the look. Ombre is probably the most commonly known look, but sombre and balayage are also very popular and quite beautiful when done correctly.

All three of these looks require a lot of knowledge and expertise to do correctly; while you will see home hair-color kits available for each of these looks, it's not easy to get professional results at home.

I recommend going to a salon and making the investment in getting your canvas professionally prepared. Then, it's up to you—you can have a stylist do your color for you, or you can take your gorgeous healthy new balayage or ombre home and light it up with the semipermanent colors of your dreams.

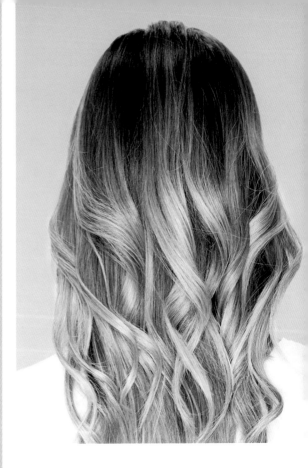

OMBRE
Ombre refers to the gradual transition from one hair color to another, in tones of natural-looking colors. Generally, an ombre dye job is darker at the roots through the mid-shaft and then gradually gets lighter from the mid-shaft to the ends. For long hair, the color technique not only is striking but also includes many different shades of color, from the darkest browns down to light platinum blond.

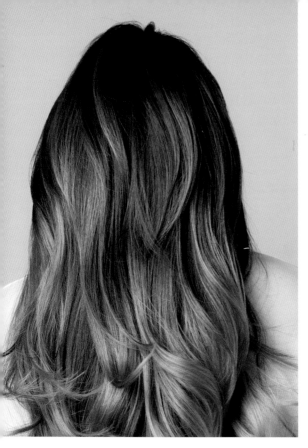

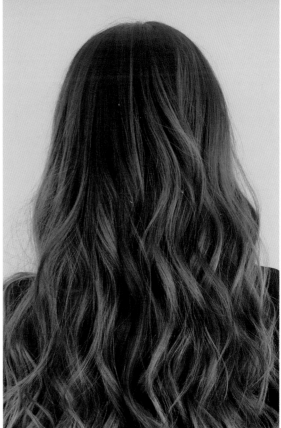

SOMBRE

Sombre hair is very similar to ombre. Sombre relies on a softer transition of color. You may not be able to tell where one shade ends and another begins if you look at the length of the hair. However, you will see a distinct difference in shades if you hold the tips up to the roots of the hair. The beauty of the style really stands out in layered cuts. A very low maintenance style, sombre is perfect for a small change in color.

BALAYAGE

Balayage is the freehand painting in which ombre and sombre trends are applied. A great balayage treatment can leave your hair looking far more natural than streaked highlights of the past. To give your hair the extra edge in coloring that can be subtle or brilliantly striking to match your personality and hair style, you can ask for balayage highlights, lowlights, ombre, or sombre style.

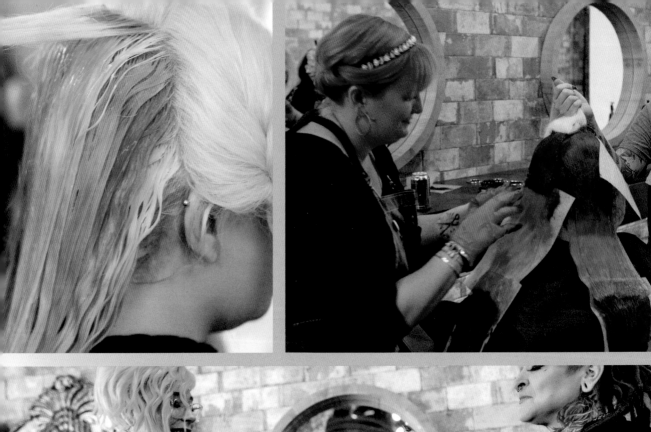

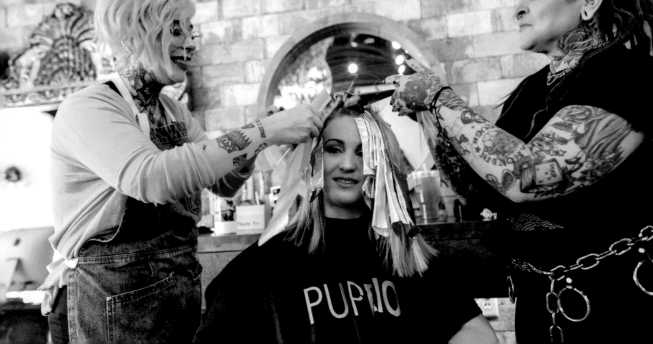

APPLYING COLOR

Now that you've learned about your hair, studied some color theory, and chosen your colors, the moment of truth has arrived—it's time to start painting your masterpiece.

Each look's instructions will walk you through the process of creating it step by step. For example, some don't need sectioning, as they're an all-over wash of color (such as the Rose Gold Sombre on page 54), or a precision free-hand design (like the Neon Rainbow Lightning Bolt on page 76). Here are some basic things to keep in mind.

SECTIONING The pointy end of your color-application brush is designed to help you make clean, precise sections. You can also use a rat-tail comb. To start, part your hair down the middle from front to nape. Then, depending on the pattern that the headsheet calls for, use the brush tip or comb to divide out sections. When we call for a 1-inch section, that means an inch along the horizontal or diagonal line. For very dense hair, you may end up with a lot more sections than for thinner hair. Always err on the side of more precise sections, because that will get you the best color saturation and help ensure you don't skip any spots.

PAINTING ON THE COLOR Whether you paint the color freehand onto a section or lay the section on foil or meche to paint is something of a personal choice, though the longer the hair and the more complex the pattern, the more it makes sense to use foil or meche (see the mermaid look, at left, which would have been almost impossible to apply freehand without making a mess of things). Hold the sections with medium tension at a low angle, and paint on enough color to fully saturate the hair.

When applying complicated color patterns where you want to be sure the colors don't bleed together, you should wait until an application of color has partially dried (a process known as "encapsulation") before applying the next color. This will take a bit longer, but the effort can really pay off.

COLOR MELTING A specific technique for applying dye, color melting is used to softly blend colors with no harsh lines. The key is to feather the spots where one color ends and the next begins, without muddying them. You can lightly blend these transition points with a fine comb, or smear them with your fingers.

PROCESSING Once the color has been applied to your whole head, follow directions for processing time. In general, that will be 20 to 30 minutes. In this case, processing literally just means letting the dye sit on your hair. Then, rinse in cool water. Don't shampoo, as this may muddy your colors.

top left: Neon Unicorn, page 64, *top right:* Magical Mermaid, p. 136, *bottom:* Lightening the canvas

AFTERCARE

Part of the fun of semipermanent color is that it's just that—not permanent. It will fade and wash out, leaving you with a canvas that's ready for your next creative inspiration. But of course you don't want your hair to fade too fast. Here's how to keep your look fresh for the maximum time.

SHAMPOO SPARINGLY Shampoo will not only strip out color; it can also muddy and blur the clean delineations of multicolor looks. Depending on your hair, some people can get away with shampooing every other day, or even less frequently, using dry shampoo in between. There are also shampoo formulations for colored hair, which are gentler.

CHILL OUT The less heat your color is exposed to, the longer it will last. In practice, that means shower (or at least rinse your hair) in the coldest water you can stand. Second to overly harsh shampoos, hot water is the biggest enemy to long-lasting hair color, so remember that every time you step into the shower.

STAY IN CONDITION Unlike shampoo, conditioner is always good for your hair. You can use tinted conditioner to keep your color fresh or even add a little bit of your dye to any conditioner (or course this only works with fairly monochromatic dye jobs . . . sadly, nobody has yet invented a rainbow-striped conditioner).

EMBRACE THE FADE Some effects only get better as they fade. Throughout this book, I've noted colors that will fade beautifully, as well as hints for getting a gorgeously lived-in look from the very start. Especially these days, with soft, melted pastels on trend, this is a great way to get the very most out of your efforts.

USE SUN PROTECTION The sun can fade your colors with too much exposure. Sometimes this can look cool, but if you want to keep a bold hot pink from turning into cotton candy, invest in sun-protectant hair spray, which also has the advantage of being moisturizing.

top: Laser Roots, page 110, *bottom:* Sunwashed Shade, page 38.

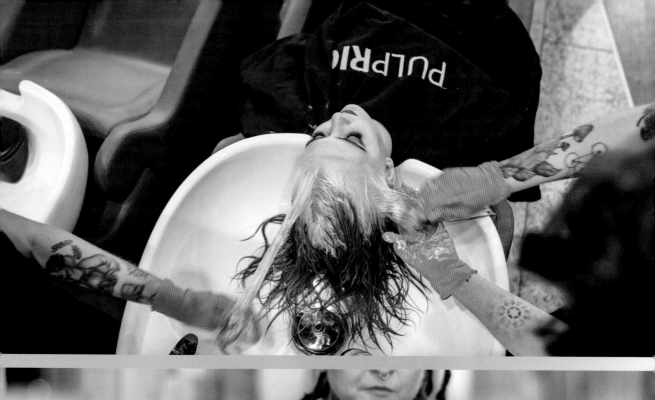
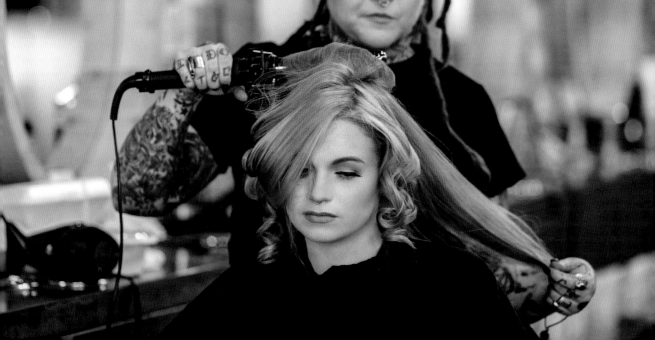

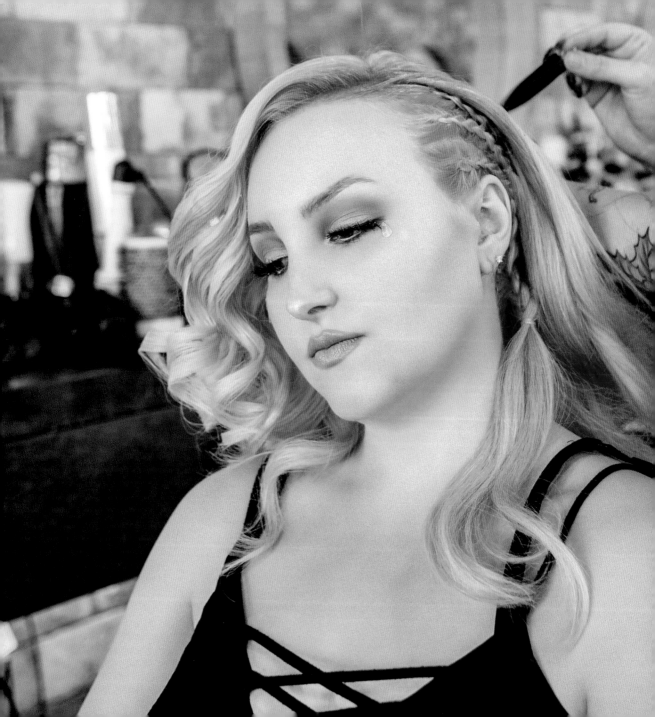

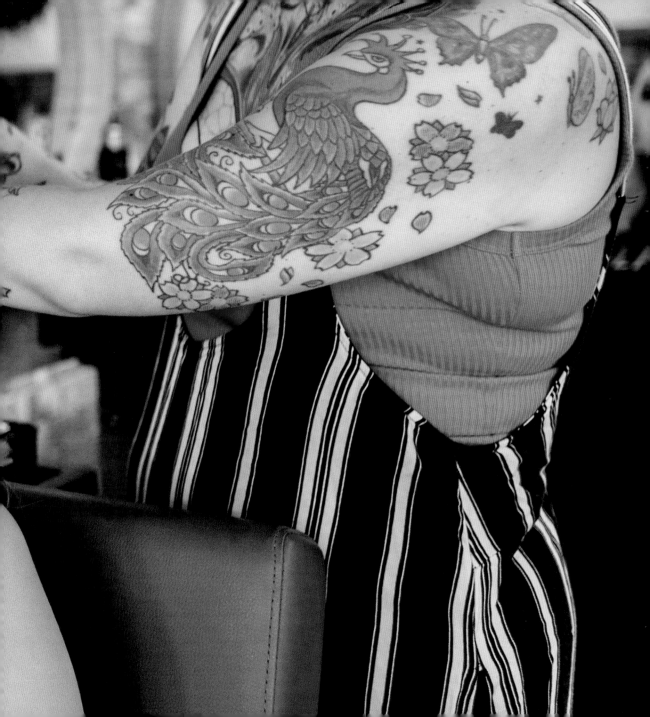

SOFT
COLORS

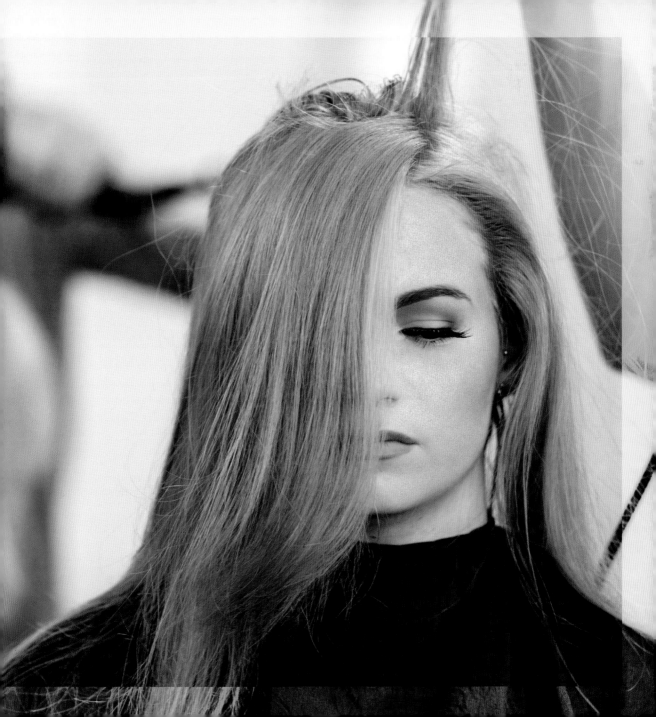

Pastel Dreamscapes

HAIR COLOR THAT RELIES ON SOFT PASTELS AND SUNWASHED SHADES IS ONE OF THOSE TRENDS THAT, IRONICALLY ENOUGH, ISN'T FADING AWAY. THE SUBTLEST OF THESE TONES ARE GREAT FOR ANYONE WHO'S JUST STARTING TO EXPERIMENT WITH COLOR OR DOESN'T WANT ANYTHING TOO INTENSE. THAT SAID, SOFT ISN'T ALWAYS SUBTLE—SOME OF THESE EFFECTS ARE REAL SHOW-STOPPERS. THERE'S NO RIGHT OR WRONG AS LONG AS YOU LOVE THE COLORS YOU'RE WORKING WITH. IF YOU WANT TO USE, SAY, A DIFFERENT ROOT FORMULA OR A BOLDER TONE FOR ONE OF THESE LOOKS, MY TUTORIALS ARE FLEXIBLE ENOUGH TO ALLOW FOR YOUR INDIVIDUAL STYLE TO SHINE.

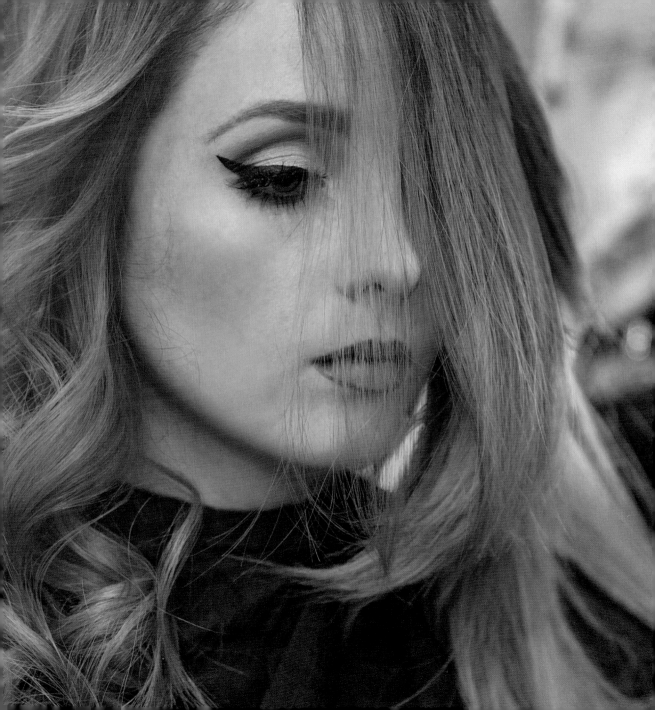

Sienna's hair needed to be lifted to a Level 9 (see the color chart on page 18).

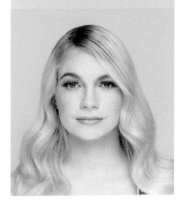

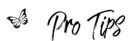

Pro Tips

For the tan formula, you can customize how neutral the color comes out—the more neutral you want it, the more light green you should add. To warm up the formula, which may be necessary if you have a warmer canvas, add more yellow or light pink.

A color melt is a technique used to blend colors together smoothly, so that they transition without any harsh breaks or divisions. For details, see page 29.

FREE-FLOATING VERTICAL COLOR MELT

SUNWASHED SHADE

The beauty of this gorgeous technique is that it offers you a lot of freedom to get creative and really personalize it depending on the colors you use and how bold you want to go. And even better, it's practically foolproof! The key is to give yourself one consistent root color, and then use the bricklay technique (see page 25) to melt the colors any way you like. They'll blend beautifully into a look that's multilayered and will transform beautifully as it fades, making for easy maintenance of the basic effects the next time you color. For Sienna's look here, my color inspiration came from a very muted bohemian mood board, inspiring the name Sunwashed Shade.

PREPARING THE CANVAS

Before applying your customized color palette, you'll want to prepare your canvas as we did for Sienna. The coloring formulations here were ones I chose specifically to complement our model's hair after it was lightened.

Sienna came in with a 2-inch natural root, which we lightened out slowly, so that her hair would stay in good condition. We lifted her to a low Level 9, and then we toned her canvas—using silver and violet toners—in order to help cancel out the warm, unnatural yellow that often comes with bleaching.

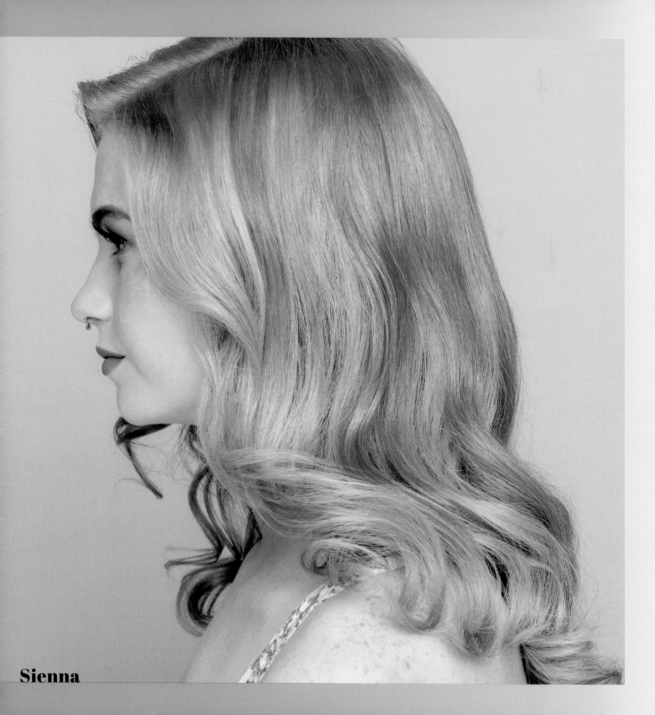

Sienna

ROOT FORMULA

1 part white conditioner + 1 part Soft Pink + 1 part Soft Purple + a bit of Light Silver

MELTING FORMULAS

Soft Blue: 1 part white conditioner + 1 part Pastel Blue + a bit of Light Silver

Soft Purple: 1 part white conditioner + 1 part Soft Purple + a bit of Light Silver

Tan: 1 part white conditioner + 1 part Neon Orange + 1 part Pale Green + 1 part Bold Yellow + 1 part Soft Pink

Soft Pink: 4 parts white conditioner + 1 part Soft Pink

Medium Lavender: 1 part Soft Purple + 1 part Deep Purple

APPLYING THE COLOR

1 The trick to a subtly lived-in look is to apply a distinct root color first, evenly all over. Apply your root formula using diagonal back sections, starting at the nape of your neck.

2 Move around your head, continuing to apply the root formula until you have even coverage on your roots.

3 After this, it gets a lot more free-form! Pick a color, any color, and start applying it in vertical panels, wherever on the head you please.

4 Apply the other color formulas as desired, melting the vertical sections into each other as you go. This look was done in a bricklay pattern, meaning that the panels of color are offset from each other. See headsheets for a visual reference.

PROCESSING

Let process at room temperature for 35 minutes, then rinse with cold water until the water runs clear.

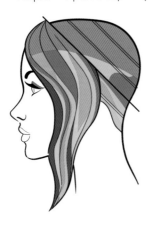
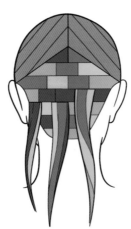

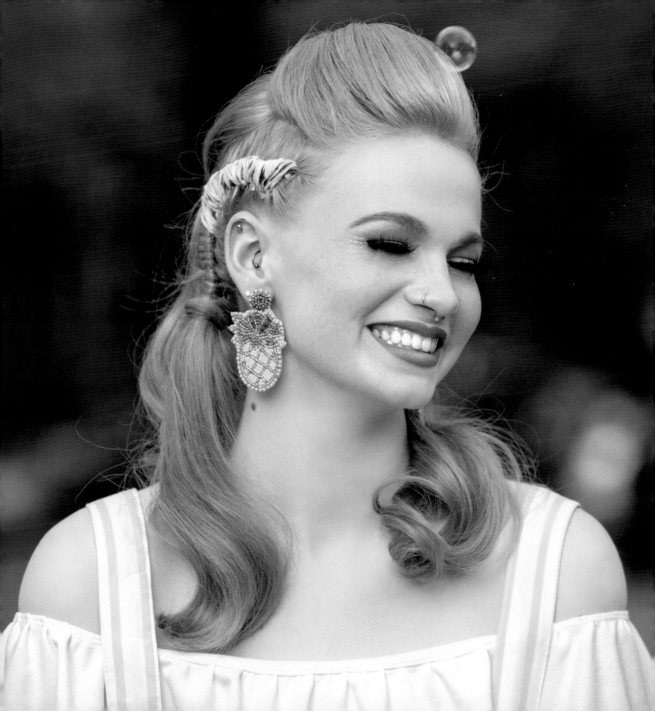

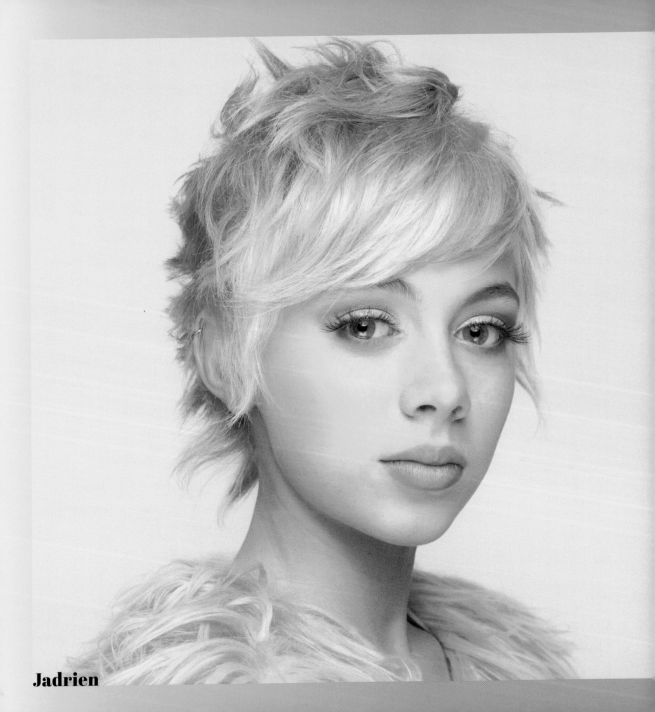

Jadrien

COLOR MELT
OPAL FLARES

This transformation uses soft, pastel pops throughout Jadrian's predominantly blonde canvas, which gave us these gorgeous, flare-like dimensions. Our goal for this look was to leave her hair 80 percent blonde, with 20 percent colorful flares throughout.

PREPARING THE CANVAS
Since we were working with a short hair cut, we applied the lightener in diagonal slices, and then color-melted our chosen shades into the surrounding hair. We started by lightening our model from root to ends, lifting her hair up to a high Level 9 and then toning it to a cool, icy blonde.

After we were done with the toner, we shampooed Jadrian, and then blow-dried her hair until it was completely dry, so that we could apply the creative colors to dry hair for greater precision and control of the individual segments.

Jadrian's hair needed to be lightened to a Level 9 (see the color chart on page 18).

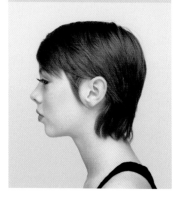

 Pro Tip

When working with shorter hair, you will want to apply colors throughout the hair while being mindful not to apply horizontal or vertical melts too harshly. Otherwise, the color can end up looking splotchy or throwing off the design of the haircut. Stay mindful of placement. With short hair, less really is more.

This technique is ideal for shorter hair, but could definitely be applied to medium or long hair as well.

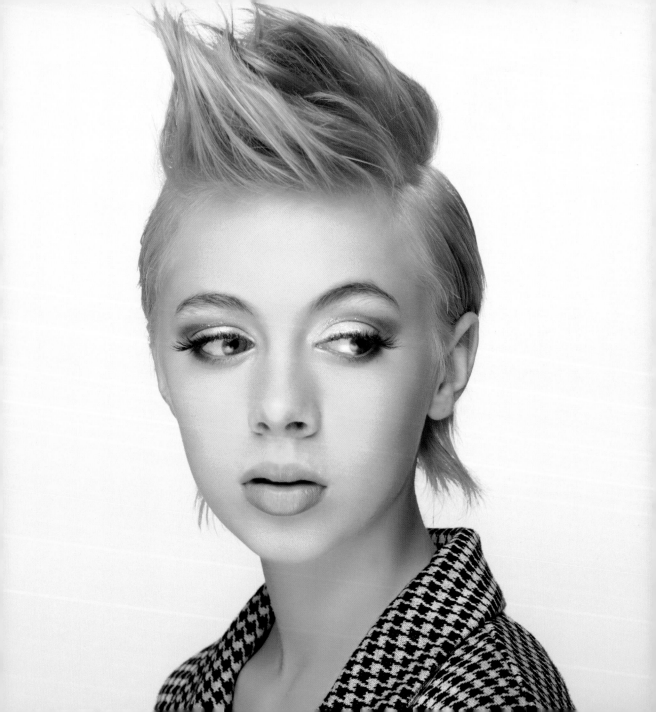

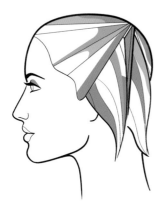

COLOR FORMULA
Melting Formulas

Light Silver: 1 part white conditioner + 1 part Light Silver

Light Pink: 1 part white conditioner + 1 part Soft Pink

Light Green: 1 part white conditioner + 1 part Electric Green

Light Blue: 1 part white conditioner + 1 part Pastel Blue

Light Purple: 1 part Light Silver + 1 part Soft Purple

APPLYING THE COLOR

1 Grab a comb to keep handy while you apply the color. That way, you can comb through the hair as or after you apply the color, in order to keep the tinted sections looking more lived in and naturally blended.

2 For this look, the colors are applied free-hand, and then melted into the hair around them. Pick a place on the hair to start and then slowly work around the head. Apply the color to patches of hair that are naturally more prominent or prone to motion, or where the hair is a little longer.

3 As you go, comb through the patches of dye and the hair around them. This will help to move the color smoothly into the hair and allow the dimensions to be more balanced and free flowing.

PROCESSING
Let process at room temperature for 30 minutes and rinse with cool water until the water runs clear.

We kept Iyanna's natural roots to avoid damaging or breaking her hair.

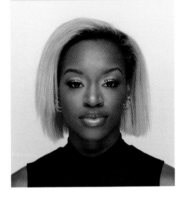

 Pro Tip

We use Pulp Riot Mercury for quite a few formulas. It's a lovely violet-based silver and a great, soft shade that helps to subtly mute the pastel colors we've chosen here. Adding it, or a similar violet-based light silver from another brand, lets you create a gorgeous, soft color palette, as in Iyanna's look.

COLOR MELT FOR SHORT HAIR

SUCCULENT HAIR

This transformation is inspired by the gorgeous iridescent colors we see in succulent plants. To achieve the look, we combined soft, muted pastels and gently melted them into each other. This fun hairstyle can also be worn down, but the way the colors blend into each other creates a wonderful, layered updo.

PREPARING THE CANVAS

Iyanna has really beautiful kinky, curly, coarse hair. It's been lightened several times before, and because of that, we decided to take precautions when doing our own lightning.

Her natural regrowth was only about 1-2 inches long, so we decided to let her natural roots create a more lived-in look. Her hair had been lightened enough times that doing so again was risky—her hair could have literally broken off in our hands!

APPLYING THE COLOR

1 Section the hair into 1-inch horizontal sections in order to apply the root formula.

2 Begin by applying your root color, starting at the crown of your head. Take a 1-inch horizontal section, apply your root formula, and then repeat that process.

3 After you've applied the root color, you may notice the color has encapsulated, forming a dry, hard shell that keeps the color from transferring to other sections. If you can wait for that, it will be it easier to apply the dye to the next sections.

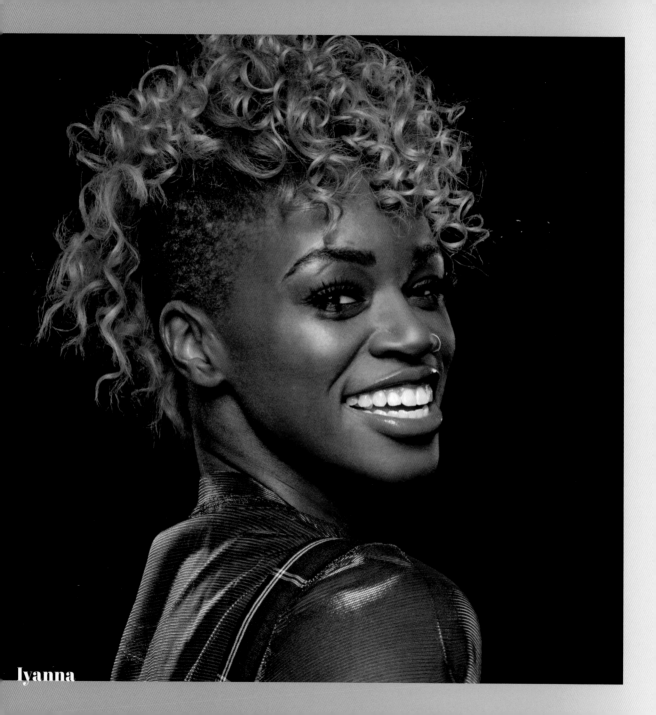

Iyanna

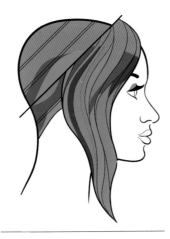

COLOR FORMULA
Root Formula
1 part Soft Pink + 1 part Fuchsia + 1 part Violet-Based Silver

Melting Formulas
Soft Mint: 1 part white conditioner + 1 part Mint + 1 part Pastel Blue

Soft Periwinkle: 1 part Soft Purple + 1 part Pastel Blue

Soft Rose: 1 part white conditioner + 1 part Soft Pink + 1 part Violet-Based Silver

4 Moving on to the melting formulas, pick one color to start with, and apply to a 1- to 2-inch section.

5 Then pick up another color and apply to a 1- to 2-inch section next to the first color block.

6 Repeat with the third dye. If you're working with a mohawk, undercut, or other hair style where you're only dyeing the hair on the top of your head, this should cover half the width of the area to be dyed.

7 Continue applying the colors to fill out the rest of that line, alternating them. As you apply the blocks of color, melt them together at the edges, so they blend well.

8 Move up or down your head from the first row of color, and start a second row—but start so that the blocks of color are offset from the first row, and the borders between them don't line up. This is called bricklay dyeing (see page 25), and it gives the hair dye a beautiful variance and dimension.

9 Continue applying different rows, offsetting each one from the last, until you have covered the desired area.

PROCESSING
Process at room temperature for 30 minutes, then rinse with cold water until the water runs clear.

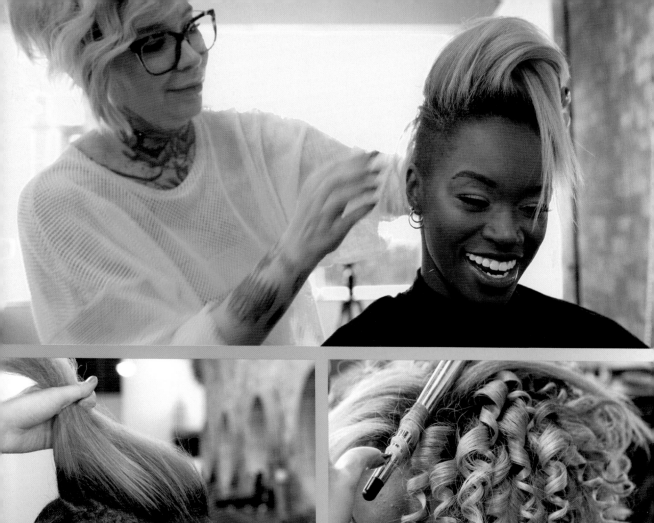
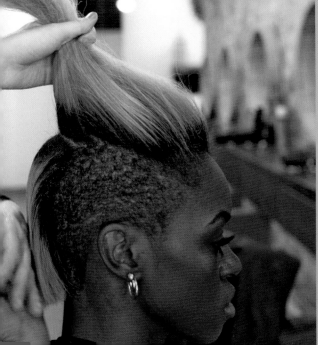
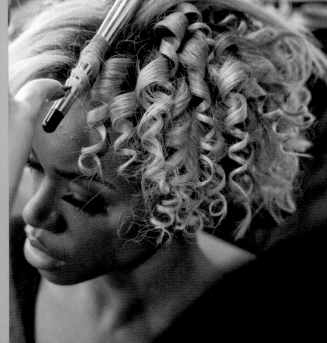

Pro Tip

This technique showcases the fact that demipermanent dyes also have creative colors—here, a rose gold toner and a pure pigment copper booster.

If you like to part your hair on the side—or anywhere other than in the center—you should customize the style by making the vertical quadrants line up with your usual parting, for a cleaner look.

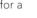

SOMBRE WITH A COLOR MELT OVERLAY

COPPER AND ROSE GOLD CRISS CROSS

This is a softer but still unique style—and one perfect for people who want to keep their hair dye low key and more professionally acceptable.

This technique is not only super easy, it's also very versatile and customizable. I call this Criss Cross because you part the hair into 4 quadrants and melt the colors together from there. The colors we chose for this transformation were Rose Gold and Copper. They both live in similar families, so although using the quadrants will make the dye pop, the colors will blend together subtly enough to have a soft (and practical!) final result.

PREPARING THE CANVAS

Kandi has naturally copper hair, which is part of why we chose this color scheme—her roots were coming in above her previous balayage, and we really wanted to build on her natural tones. Working in the same color family as her roots also makes for easier maintenance as her roots grow out. We didn't quite keep her root its natural color, though—instead, we made it a deep mahogany, to give the look more depth.

Kandi's natural roots are a Level 7 true copper, and the Level 8 and 9 on the rest of her hair kept the canvas beautifully warm. When working with warm tones like coppers and rose golds, you need to decide if you want to pretone the hair to soften the vibrancy—if you're like me and want to utilize the vibrancy, you'll skip the toning and just deposit your colors.

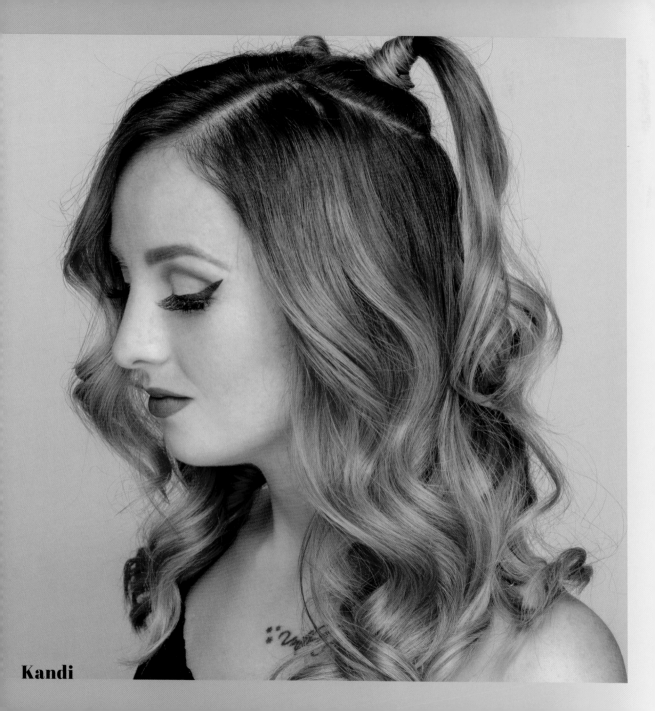

Kandi

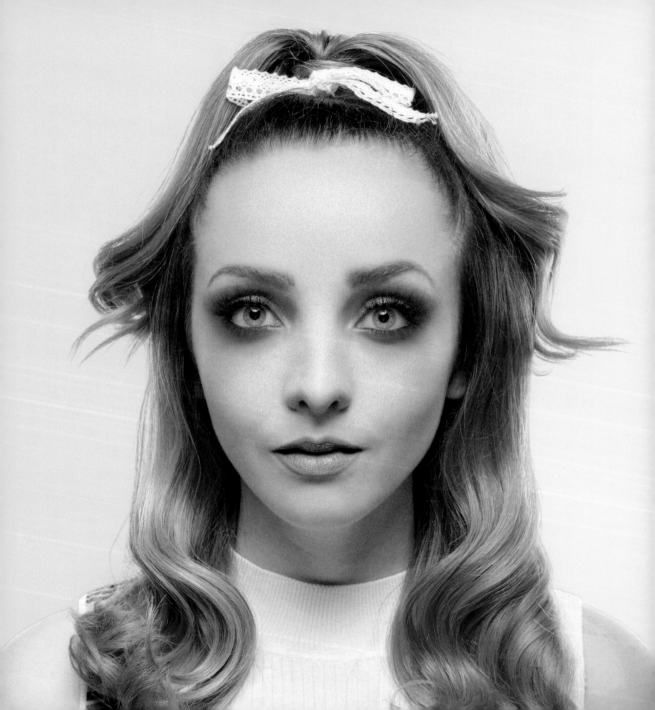

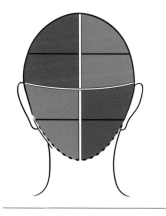

COLOR FORMULA
Root Formula
Permanent dark red-brown hair dye

Quadrant Formulas
Rose Gold: 1 part High Speed Toner in Rose Gold + 2 parts 6 volume developer

Copper: 1 part Demipermanent Copper + 2 parts 6 volume developer

APPLYING THE COLOR

1 Section your hair into 4 quadrants. Do this by parting your hair twice: First vertically, from the nape of your neck to your forehead. Then horizontally, from the top of one ear, over the top of your head, to the top of the other.

2 Clip the extra 3 sections so that they stay separate and, starting on whichever section you'd like, apply the root formula to the first 2 inches of your hair.

3 Work the root formula into the other 3 quadrants.

4 Next, take Quadrant 1, split it in half horizontally, and apply the Copper Formula to each half, from roots to ends.

5 Apply the formulas to the other 3 quadrants using the following pattern, being sure to blend the Quadrant Formulas into the Root Formula:
Quadrant 2. Right front section = Rose Gold Formula
Quadrant 3. Left back section = Rose Gold Formula
Quadrant 4. Right back section = Copper Booster Formula

PROCESSING
Allow the color to process at room temperature for 35 minutes and then lightly shampoo the hair in cool water. Shampoo is used here, unlike in many of our other looks, because you need it to get out the demipermanent dye.

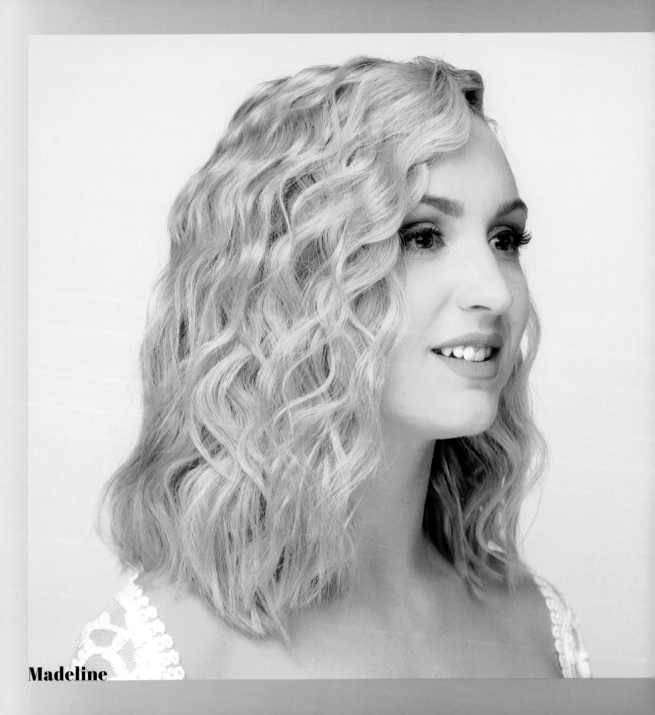

Madeline

SOMBRE WITH A ROSE GOLD TONER AND
A BACK-TEASING FOILAGE

ROSE GOLD SOMBRE

This fun concept and technique is all about creating a more subtle, low-maintenance look built on top of a sombre—a bolder version of the classic ombre. The contrast between the blonde and the natural roots is less harsh, meaning the look can give really bold blonde dimensions that are more seamlessly melted together. Overall, this softens a natural root without the high maintenance of traditional highlights.

Sombres work with more shades and tones throughout the hair, adding high contrast, plus more dimensions closer to the root.

PREPARING THE CANVAS

Madeline had preexisting highlights and a balayage done on her hair, so a lot of it was already lightened. For our own lightening, we back-teased the hair before applying foils in order to leave a small bit of her natural root, while also creating finely woven highlights that would break up her natural root color and blend in bright, lived-in highlights. Doing so left Madeline's hair the perfect canvas for our rose gold.

After lightening, we applied two different toners—one that was an icy silver and one that was a rose gold—to help support and bring out her rose gold more. We let the toner process for 15 minutes, then shampooed and towel-dried.

Adding a few drops of a mint green color (we used Pulp Riot Seaglass) helps make sure that your pink isn't too pink. Pastel greens can be great for softly diluting formulas, which makes them lighter and also cools them down, neutralizing and softening them.

COLOR FORMULA
Overlay Formula
1 part white conditioner +
1 part Soft Pink + a few
drops of Mint

Rose Gold is a lighter color—and the lighter the color, the quicker it will fade with each wash. So sometimes it's a good idea to tone the hair as close to the color you're going to dye it to, and then layer a second coat on with semipermanent hair dye—which is what we did.

APPLYING THE COLOR

1   Make sure that your hair has been toned, rinsed, and partially towel-dried. You want to make sure to apply the Overlay Formula to damp hair.

2   Take your overlay formula and start painting over the highlights. Since such a light formula will only anchor to prelightened hair, applying the color is easy—the anchoring stops you from messing up!

3   Continue painting on the overlay formula. Using horizontal sectioning is ideal for helping you get all the highlighted areas of your hair.

4   Check to make sure you've covered all of the lightened areas of your hair and that you've achieved a nice, even saturation.

5   If you like the sombre effect as is, you can actually leave off the overlay formula and just use the rose gold toner to achieve your desired color.

PROCESSING
Let process until you have reached your desired shade of rose gold—that should be anywhere from 5 minutes to 30 minutes. Then rinse with cold water until the water runs clear.

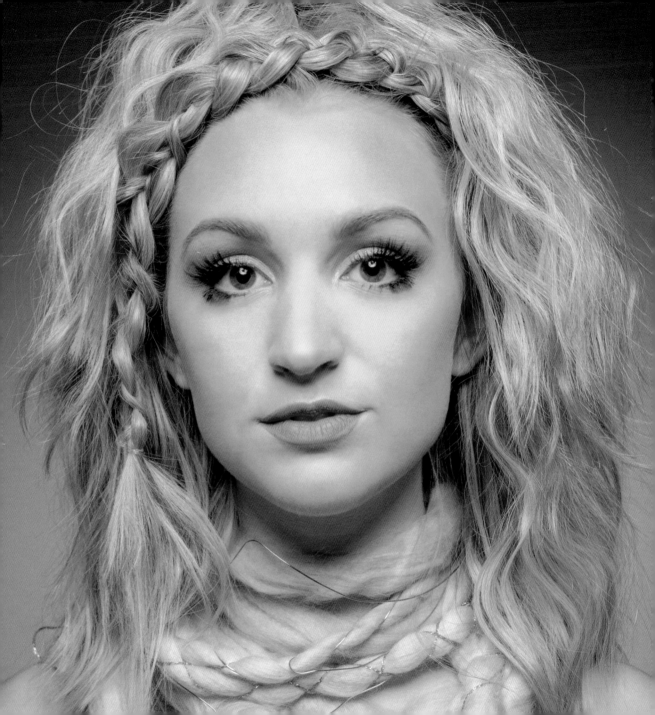

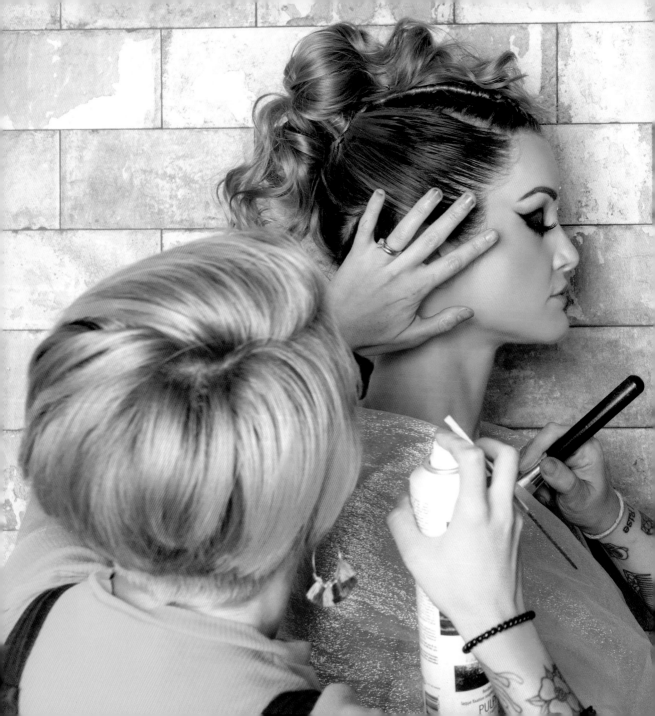

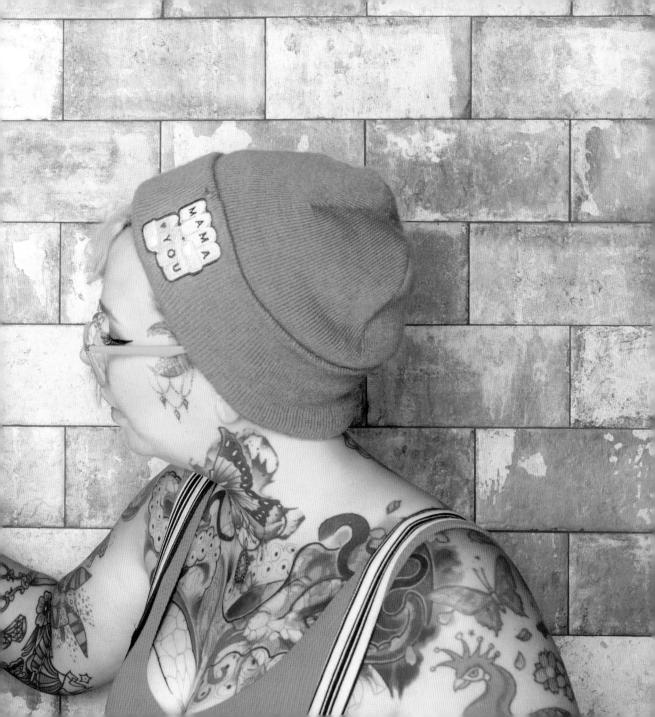

OVER THE
RAINBOW

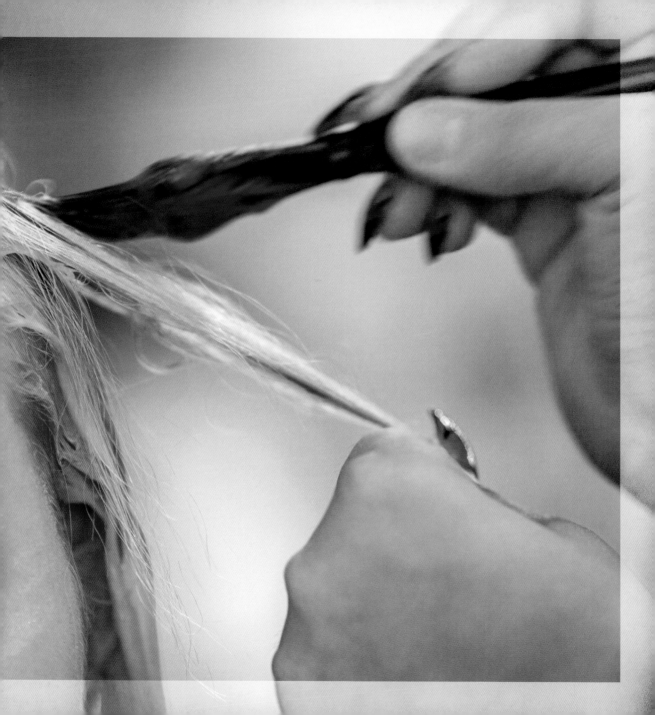

Full-Spectrum Fabulous

IF YOU'VE EVEN CASUALLY BROWSED YOUR
FAVORITE HAIR DYE BRANDS ONLINE, LET ALONE
CHECKED OUT THE AISLES AND AISLES OF
SEMIPERMANENT COLORS AVAILABLE AT YOUR
LOCAL BEAUTY STORE, YOU KNOW THAT YOU HAVE
THE ENTIRE RAINBOW (AND MORE!) TO CHOOSE
FROM. AND IF YOU CAN'T CHOOSE JUST ONE
(OR TWO . . . OR THREE) COLORS? NO PROBLEM!
THIS CHAPTER TAKES A TRIP OVER THE RAINBOW
TO BRING YOU COLOR-DRENCHED STYLES THAT
DEFINITELY AREN'T IN KANSAS ANYMORE. FROM
SHIMMERING PASTELS TO VIVID NEONS, YOU'LL
FIND A FULL SPECTRUM OF LUXURIOUS LOOKS
HERE THAT WILL BRIGHTEN ANY DAY.

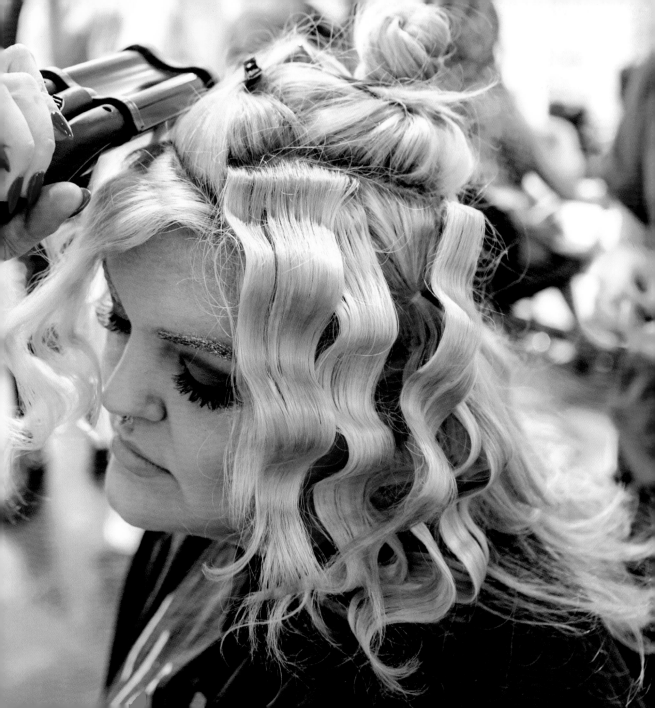

Olivia's hair and roots were bleached to a Level 10 (see the color chart on page 18).

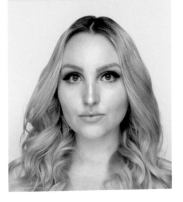

Pro Tip

In an ideal world you'd have a friend or family member there to lend a hand when you need to color the back of your head—but if you're on your own, don't worry! Just work very carefully and meticulously. Have a hand mirror in reach, and check your progress frequently in your bathroom mirror, using the hand mirror to reflect the back of your head. If brushing dye onto hair you can't see feels awkward, try using your (gloved!) fingers to apply it instead.

RAINBOW ROOTS

NEON UNICORN

For the fantasy hair of your dreams, try pairing a soft pastel overall color with vibrant rainbow roots. Painting the roots with alternating neon pastel tones creates a really captivating focal point and a soft punch of long-lasting color.

PREPARING THE CANVAS

Olivia's canvas needed to be lifted all the way to Level 10 to get the most out of these pastel tones.

APPLYING THE COLOR

1   It's important that you apply your rainbow colors in the same order all over your head. The neon pastel rainbow follows the basic color spectrum, using neon pastel pink, peach, yellow, mint, blue, and lilac, in that order.

2   **Neon Pastel Pink:** Starting at the nape of your neck, take a 1-inch horizontal section of hair and paint Neon Pastel Pink onto a two-inch length from the root down.

3   Next, apply your All Over Formula to the rest of the section, painting it from where your pink root ends all the way down to the ends. Melt the two dyes together where they meet (see page 29).

4   **Neon Pastel Peach:** Take a new 1-inch horizontal section of hair, right above the section you just painted, and apply two inches of Neon Pastel Peach starting at the root. Apply the

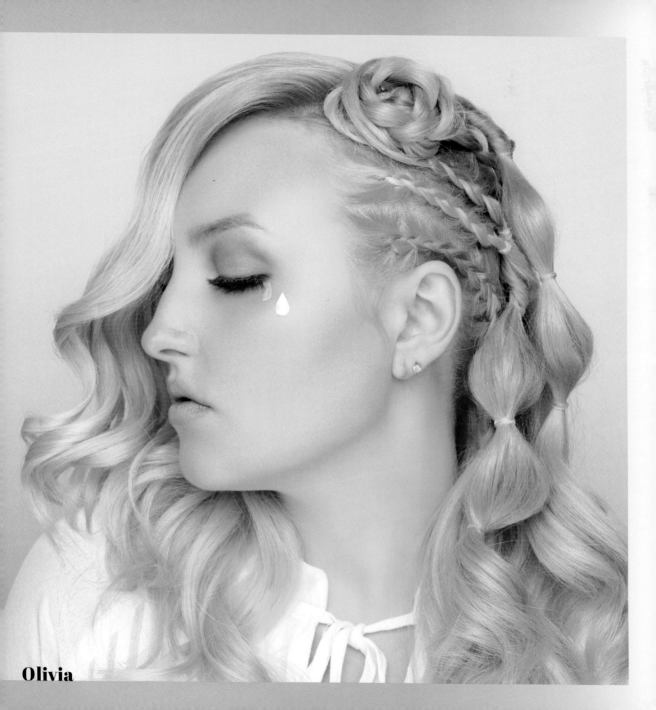

Olivia

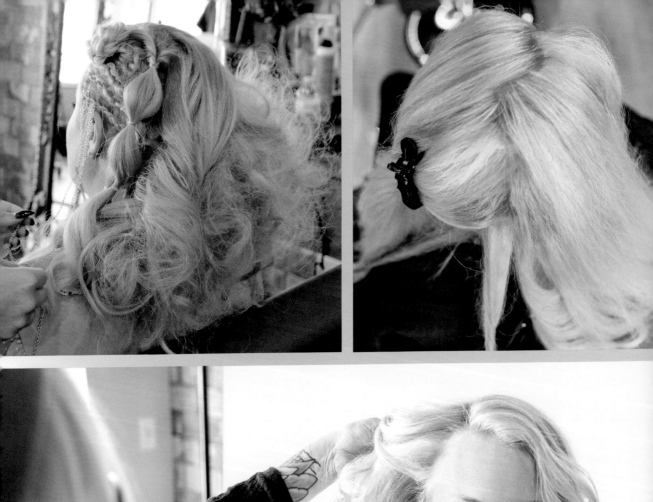
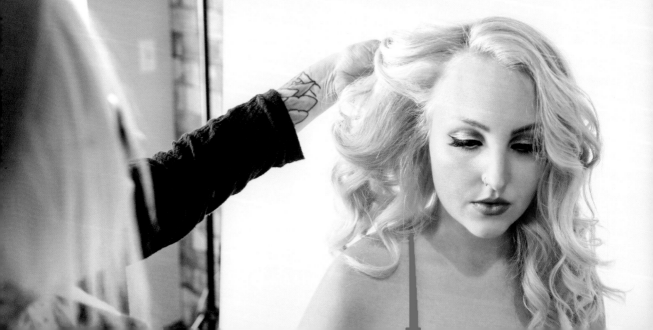

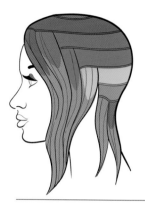

COLOR FORMULA
Neon Pastel Formulas

Pink: 1 part white conditioner + 1 part Neon Pink + 1 part Pastel Pink

Peach: 1 part white conditioner + 1 part Pastel Pink + 1 part Neon Orange

Yellow: 1 part white conditioner + 1 part Bold Yellow

Mint: 1 part white conditioner + 1 part Mint + ¼ part Neon Green

Blue: 1 part white conditioner + 1 part Pastel Blue + ¼ part Neon Blue

Lilac: 1 part white conditioner + 1 part Lilac + ¼ part Neon Blue + ¼ part Pastel Pink

All Over Formula
1 part white conditioner + 1 part Soft Pink

All Over Formula to the rest, blending it into the peach as you go. Once you finish, let this section gently lay on top of the just-colored hair below it.

5 **Neon Pastel Yellow:** Now take the another 1-inch section and follow the same steps as above, this time applying 2 inches of Neon Pastel Yellow, followed by the All Over Formula.

6 **Neon Pastel Mint:** Follow the same steps with the Neon Pastel Mint, applying as above.

7 **Neon Pastel Blue:** Next, do the same with Neon Pastel Blue, again applying for 2 inches and then melting thoroughly into the All Over Formula.

8. **Neon Pastel Lilac:** Repeat the same steps with the Neon Pastel Lilac Formula—this will complete your first rainbow!

The rainbow should go all the way from the nape of your neck to the crown of your head. You may need to adjust how much hair you take into the last few sections to make it even out.

Once the back of your head is complete, do the sides of your head, one at a time. Be sure to start with the same color each time, so that each forms a continual ring around your head.

PROCESSING
Let process at room temperature for 30 minutes and rinse with cold water until the water runs clear.

Sarah's hair is lightened to a Level 10 (see the color chart on page 18).

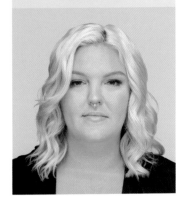

 Pro Tip

Although you don't need to if you don't want to, this is a look where you can definitely benefit from using foil or meche strips (see glossary) to isolate the different sections and keep the colors from cross-contaminating. If you don't want to use them, though, you should definitely wait for each section to encapsulate, or harden, before laying the next one on top of it. This will prevent the dye from transferring across sections.

COLOR MELT

RAINBOW GLAZE

This lovely look is all about the pastels, and the technique used here will let you create a seamless, radiant rainbow glaze with those soft tones. This is a fun, easy, creative way to give your hair a soft rainbow effect, which is both extremely beautiful and also an unusual take on the traditional rainbow. Instead of red, orange, yellow, green, blue, indigo, and violet, this rainbow's pastel spectrum shimmers from pink to peach to yellow to green to blue, and finally to lilac.

The formulas can be customized a bit, depending on the amount of white conditioner you use to dilute the dye and create your pastels. To avoid wasting product, start with a small amount of conditioner in each mixing bowl. Add a dash of color, and mix well. To intensify the color, add more dye; for a softer pastel, add more conditioner.

PREPARING THE CANVAS

For the pastels to really glow, Sarah's hair needed to be at the lightest level, Level 10. A very light canvas will keep the colors bright and their tones pure, which is perfect for the end effect this technique will give you: tiny, soft sheets of color that shimmer and almost seem to softly reflect each other. You won't know where one color ends and one begins.

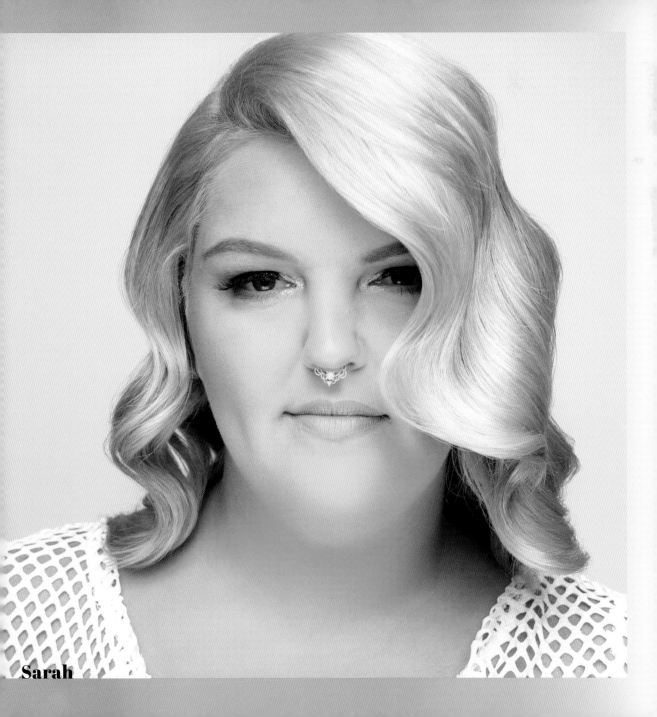

Sarah

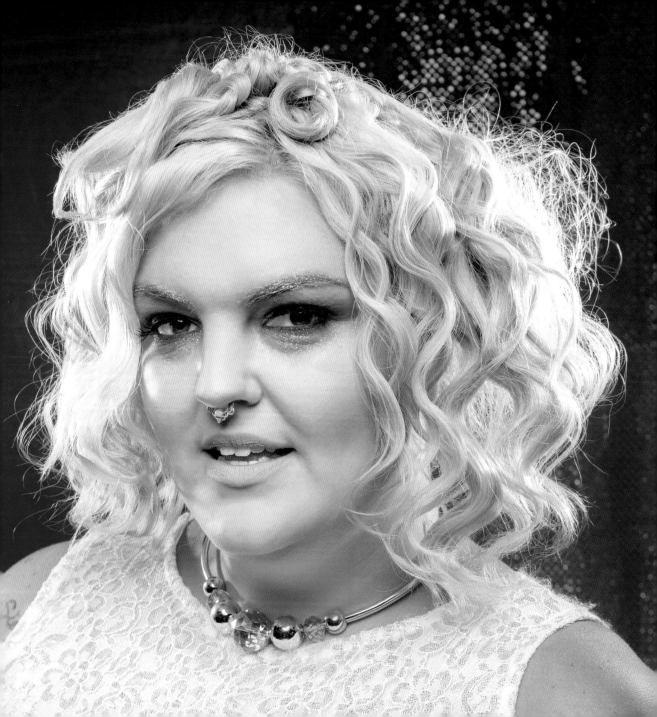

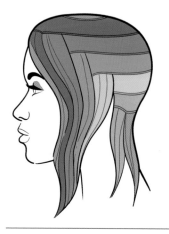

COLOR FORMULA

Pastel Pink: 4 parts white conditioner + 1 part Pastel Pink

Pastel Peach: 4 parts white conditioner + 1 part Pastel Pink + 1 part Soft Orange

Pastel Yellow: 4 parts white conditioner +1 part Soft Yellow

Pastel Green: 4 parts white conditioner + 1 part Green

Pastel Blue: 4 parts white conditioner + 1 part Pastel Blue

Pastel Lilac: 4 parts white conditioner + 1 part Pastel Lilac

APPLYING THE COLOR:

1 **Pastel Pink:** Starting at the nape of your neck, take a 1-inch horizontal section and paint your pink formulation from the roots all the way down to the ends.

2 **Pastel Peach:** Now, take the next 1-inch section, which should be above the one you've just painted. Apply your peach color from root to ends, and lay it gently on top of the pink section.

3 **Pastel Yellow:** Follow the above steps, this time using Pastel Yellow for the next 1-inch section; lay the finished section gently on top of the completed peach section below it.

4 **Pastel Green:** Paint the next section using the Pastel Green.

5 **Pastel Blue:** For the next 1-inch section, repeat using blue.

6 **Pastel Lilac:** Lastly, apply your lilac to the next section, to complete your first rainbow.

Repeat the rainbow pattern until you've finished the back of your head. Do the sides next, and finish with the top.

When working on the sides, be sure to start with the same color each time, so that the section framing your face and temples will match the color at the same height in the back.

PROCESSING

Let process at room temperature for 30 minutes and rinse with cold water until the water runs clear.

Meghan's natural hair is a Level 6 (see the color chart on page 18).

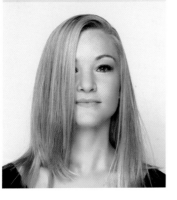

 Pro Tip

In many cases, there's no major advantage to using meche over foil. This look, however, is different for a number of reasons. The color-pattern "shine lines" are delicate and need to be offset in a bricklay pattern. For these reasons, the ability to see at a glance what colors are applied to each section makes life a lot easier. The more precise your sectioning and painting, the better this look will be in the end.

HOLOGRAM HAIR
ABALONE SHELL

Hologram hair adds smoky muted tones and pops of neon pastels to a beautiful blonde canvas. It's a unique color effect that has been sweeping the hair industry, managing to be timeless, trendy, *and* customizable.

PREPARING THE CANVAS

Meghan came in with virgin Level 6 hair, and we lightened her twice, in back-to-back sessions, so that we could bring her hair all the way up to a high Level 10, the lightest her hair could go.

Next, we needed to tone her canvas to an even icy blonde from root to end. We took a DIY approach, taking some white conditioner and making it into a custom toner by adding a splash of light purple and some light silver semipermanent color. The right toner will vary from person to person, depending on where the hair started and what end result you desire. Leave it on until the hair is toned to your satisfaction, anywhere from 5 to 25 minutes. Rinse in cold water and blow the hair completely dry.

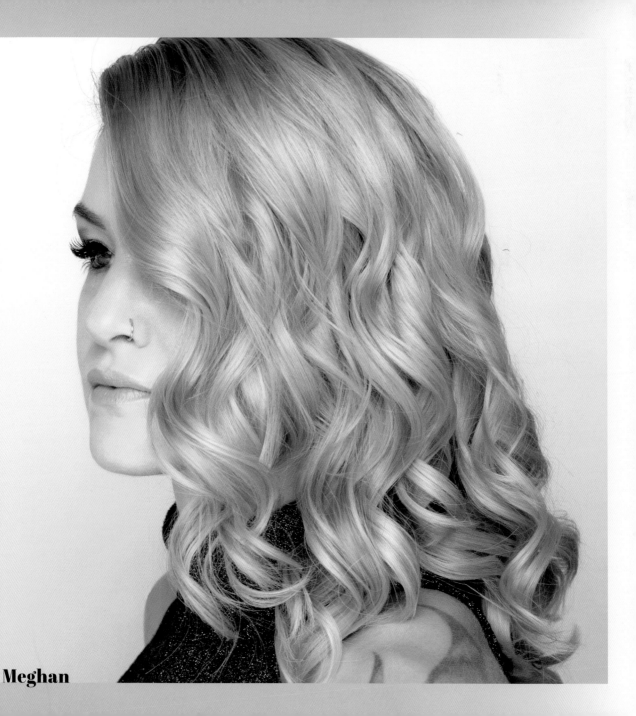

Meghan

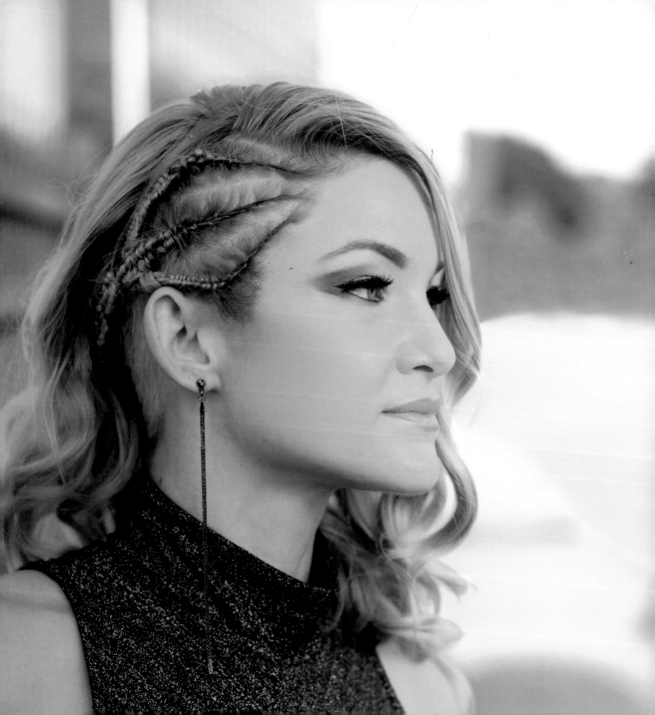

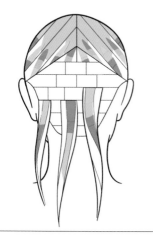

COLOR FORMULA
Root Formula
1 part Light Silver + 1 part Soft Purple + 1 part Medium Silver

First Pattern
Yellow: Bold Yellow

Pink: 1 part white conditioner + 1 part Soft Pink

Green: 1 part white conditioner + 1 part Mint Green

Purple: 1 part white conditioner + 1 part Soft Purple

Second Pattern
Green: Electric Green

Blue: 1 part white conditioner + 1 part Soft Blue

Yellow: Bold Yellow

Pink: 1 part white conditioner + 1 part Soft Pink

APPLYING THE COLOR

1 Mix up the root formula until you get a beautiful, rich silver, and then literally smudge the color onto your roots. Apply it to about the first inch or so all over your head.

2 The hologram effect is achieved by interweaving two repeating colormelt patterns offset in a bricklay pattern. Starting at the back of the head, take a diagonal back parting, and clip the rest of the hair out of your way.

3 Now take a 1-inch sub-section and place it on a strip of foil or meche. Apply your first pattern to this section, dabbing on just about a quarter inch of each color to make an inch-long "shine line" of Yellow, followed by Pink, then Green, then Purple. Use a comb or your fingers to melt the colors together, carefully blurring each transition.

4 Following the offset bricklay pattern, apply the second pattern to the next section: one quarter inch strip of Green, followed by the same amount of Blue, Yellow, and Pink to form the second shine line. Melt the colors together as you did with the first pattern.

5 Continue working around your head, making sure your patterns remain offset from each other, so the borders between them don't line up. Leave room for the different patterns to dance around and into the blonde canvas.

PROCESSING
Process at room temperature for 30 minutes, then rinse with cold water until the water runs clear.

Christian's natural roots
are a Level 5 (see the color
chart on page 18).

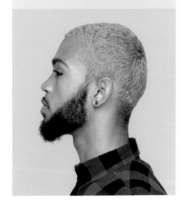

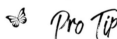
Pro Tip

Lightener works more quickly
when heated, and your head is
a good source of heat, which
explains why bleach lifts color
from your roots more quickly than
from the rest of your hair. Since
Christian had such a small natural
regrowth area to lighten, we didn't
have to be aggressive about it.
We also wanted to be mindful
of his preexisting color, because
applying lightener over an area
that's already been lightened can
cause damage.

FREEHAND PAINTING

NEON RAINBOW LIGHTNING BOLT

Short hair can be a lot of fun, providing a great canvas on which
to express your creativity. I was inspired to free-hand a colorful
lightning bolt for Christian, and it worked out even better than I
imagined with his hair's beautiful, wavy texture.

PREPARING THE CANVAS

Christian came in with hair that had been lightened before,
which presented us with the perfect canvas for a bold, warm
color palette. To start, we decided to lighten his hair just a bit
more, to not only give ourselves an all-over lighter canvas, but
also to lift his natural roots, which had grown out to about a
quarter inch since the last time he'd bleached his hair.

Processing times will vary depending on how many levels of lift
you are trying to achieve, and what can be done safely without
damaging the hair. In Christian's case, our goal was to lift his
natural Level 5 roots up 4 levels, to a Level 9, to really make the
rainbow colors pop.

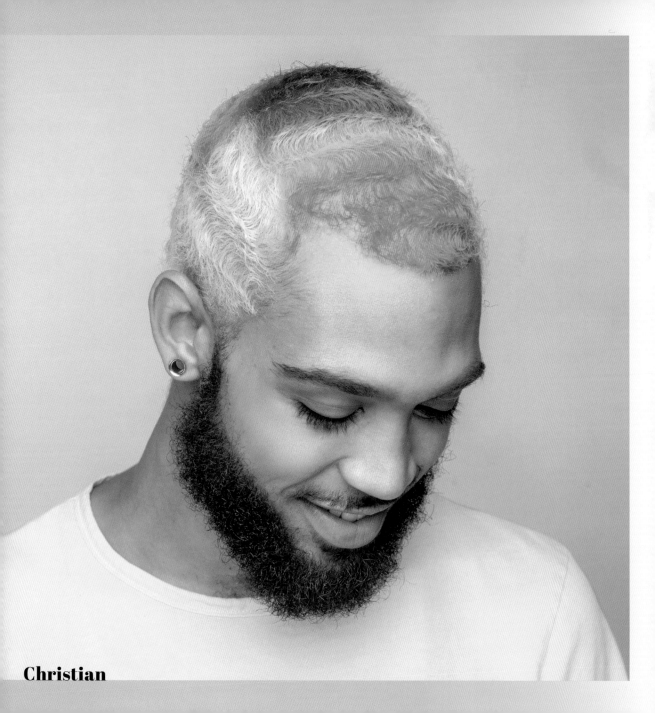

Christian

COLOR FORMULA
Base Formula
Bold Yellow

Rainbow Formulas
Neon Red: 1 part white
conditioner + 1 part Bold Red +
1 part Neon Orange

Orange: Neon Orange

Yellow: Bold Yellow

Neon Green: 1 part Electric
Green + 1 part Pale Yellow +
2 drops of Deep Teal

Neon Blue: 1 Part Pastel Blue +
2 drops of Vibrant Blue

Neon Purple: 1 part Soft Purple
+ 1 part Fuchsia

APPLYING THE COLOR

1 Figure out where you want to place your lightning bolt.

2 Trace the outline of your design with a white eyeliner pencil, which is a great tool for drawing designs on close-shaved hair, as it will come out completely when you rinse your hair.

3 Using the pencil, sketch the outlines for each block of color, making sure they are proportional.

4 Starting at the front of your head, paint the dye onto each section of the rainbow pattern, moving backwards down your head towards the nape.

5 Make sure to wash your dye brush in between color blocks so that the neons stay separate and bright.

6 After you've applied each block, melt the dye very slightly into the color before it, feathering just a little at the border between the colors to keep the transition looking smooth.

7 Once you're done with the lightning bolt, take the dye you picked for the rest of your hair (here, we chose Bold Yellow) and paint it on, being careful around the edges of your design. Bring the base color right up to the outline of your lightning bolt, but don't melt them together.

PROCESSING
Let process at room temperature for 35 minutes and rinse with cold water until the water runs clear. Coarse hair may require more through rinsing, but it's still important to avoid shampoo—otherwise the colors will bleed.

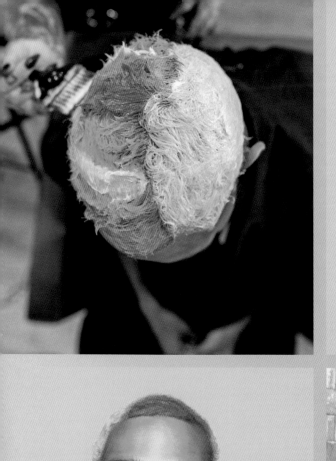
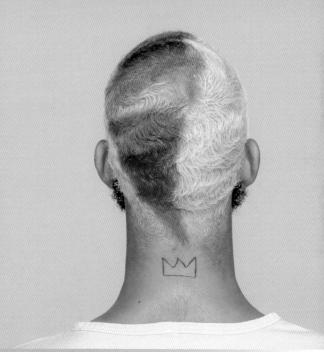
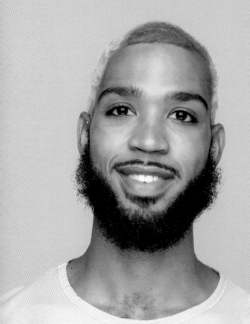
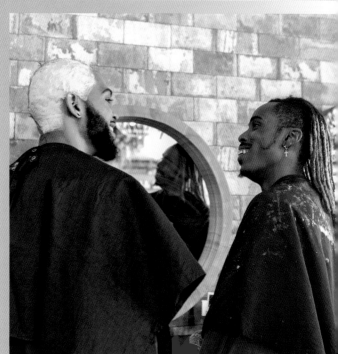

Pro Tip

Be very precise when sectioning your hair at the very beginning. Clean, intentional sections will keep your tractor beam neat and crisp looking. While painting the vertical sections, tap a little bit of the color mixture on first, and be careful not to let it bleed onto the sections in front or behind it.

You can also use your fingers to help saturate the hair completely, working the color in from root too ends. Saturation is key to good effects with any creative color; my secret is to work my brush from side to side to help cover every hair so that none of the underlying blonde remains.

TRACTOR BEAM

NEON PRISM LIGHTS

The tractor beam technique is a perfect way to add multiple vibrant pops of color all over your head. In this case, we started with a silvery gray base, and then worked in sections of diluted neons using pinwheel sectioning. This look is not only very versatile, but it appears almost ever-changing, thanks to the way the colors seem to move and flow. This makes styling a lot of fun, as your hair can look totally different from day to day depending on where you part it and whether you wear it up or down. Have some fun, play around, and see what you can do with your colors!

PREPARING THE CANVAS

Kierstin had blonde highlights on her ends when she came in, so we started by lightening her roots and color-correcting the ends to remove any brassy tones. Once she reached a consistent Level 9 across her whole head, we used a purple shampoo to pre-tone and get rid of any lingering yellow undertones. We then blow dried her until she was 100 percent dry, and proceeded to section her hair. Then the fun began!

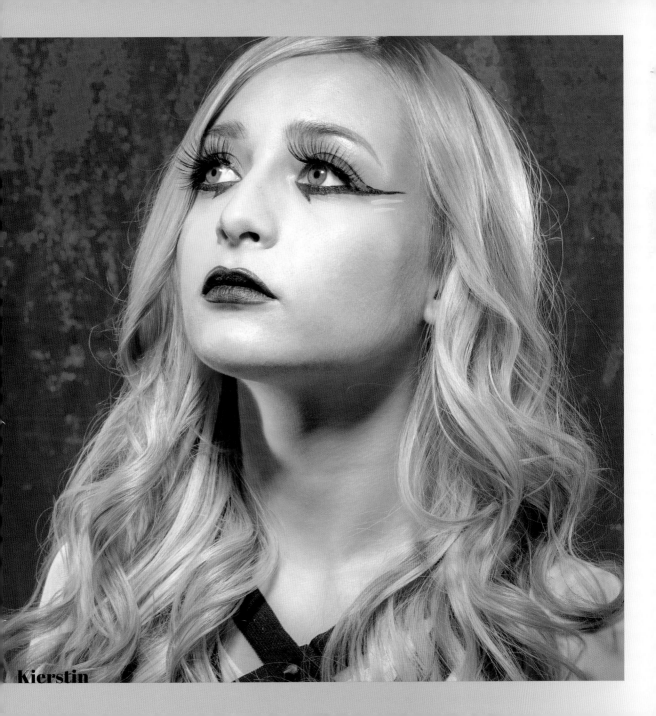

Kierstin

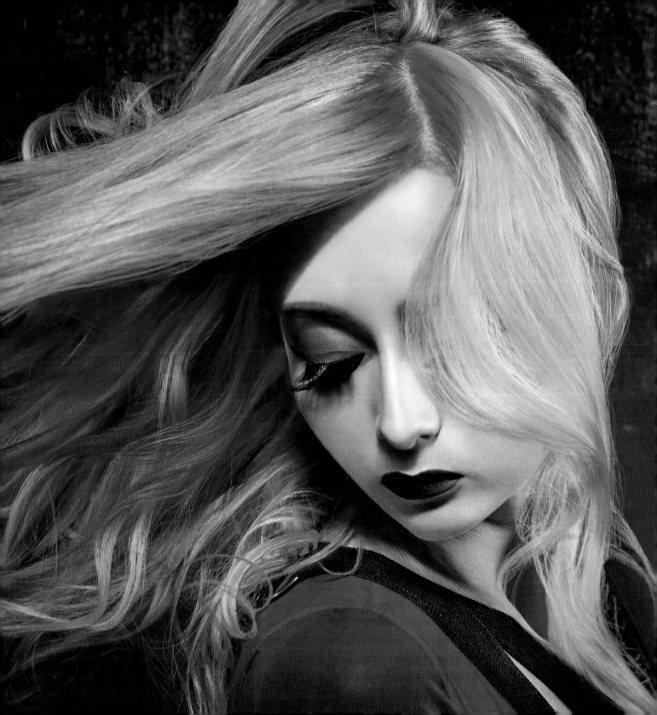

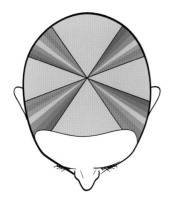

COLOR FORMULA
Base Formula
1 part white conditioner +
1 part Light Silver + a few drops
of Soft Purple

Rainbow Stripe Formulas
Pink: 1 part white conditioner
+ 1 part Neon Pink + a few
drops of Dark Pink

Orange: Neon Orange

Yellow: Lemon Yellow + a few
drops of Neon Yellow

Green: 1 part white conditioner
+ 1 part Neon Green

Blue: 1 part white conditioner
+ 1 part Powder Blue + 2 drops
Neon Blue

APPLYING THE COLOR

1 Divide your hair into 8 vertical pinwheel sections with your crown as the center of the pinwheel. Make sure that all of the sections are the same in size and density.

2 Next, paint 4 opposing sections with the Base Formula. For Kiersten, I chose to paint the middle front and back sections and the sections over her ears with the silver formulation.

3 The other 4 sections will be painted with fine rainbow stripes. Starting at the crown of the head, take a one-inch section and place it on foil or meche.

4 Start by painting a stripe of Pink at the edge of the section, from crown to ends. Next to that, paint an Orange stripe, doing your best to match the first stripe's width and color saturation. Next, paint a Yellow stripe, then a Green one, then Blue to complete the section. Carefully lay it down on the hair beneath.

5 Take up your next subsection and repeat this process, continuing until every quadrant is either base silver or rainbow striped. Make sure each color and section ends up at the same level of saturations, so that no one color ends up overpowering another.

PROCESSING
Let process at room temperature for 25 minutes, then rinse in cold water until the water runs clear.

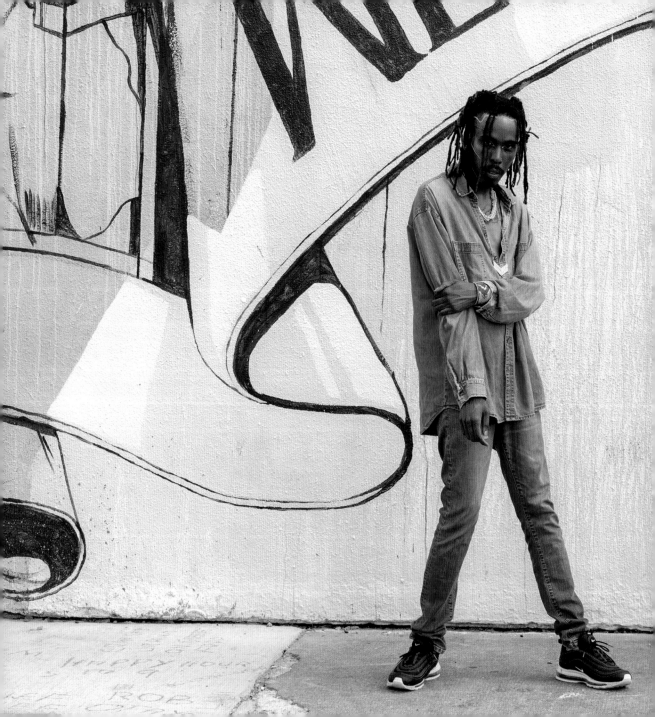

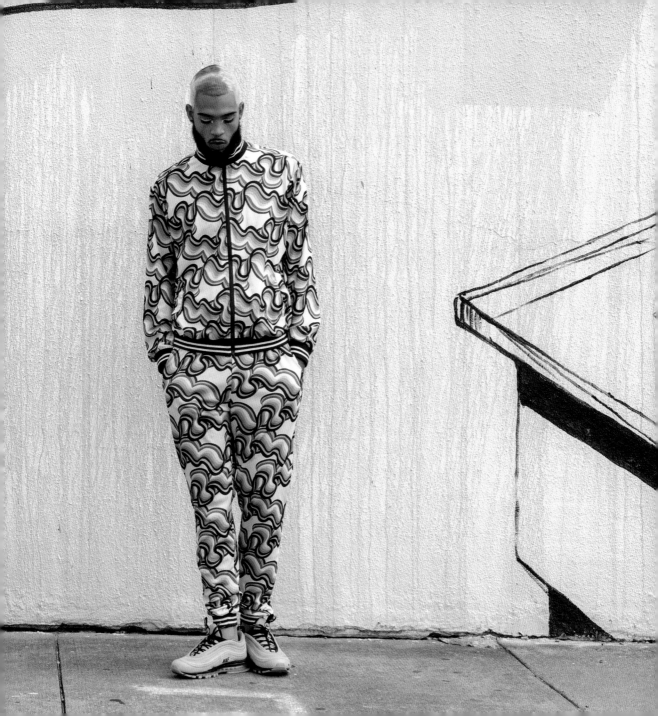

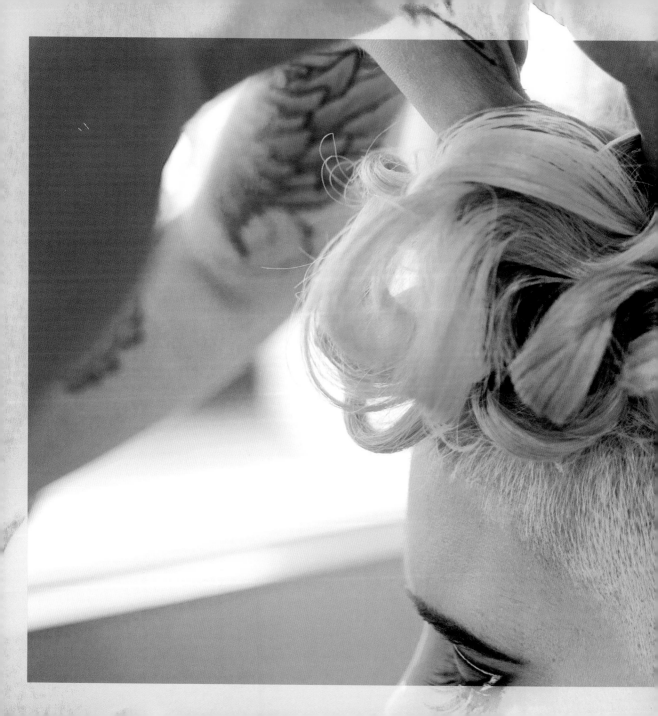

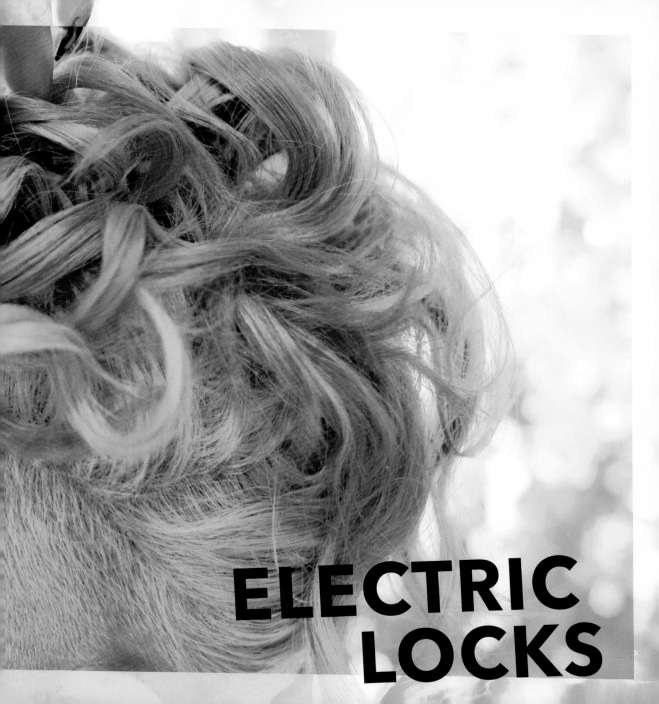

ELECTRIC
LOCKS

A Bolt from the Blue

IF YOU'RE READY FOR A BIG, BOLD LOOK, TODAY'S

COLORS CAN GIVE YOU EYE-POPPING EFFECTS

THAT RANGE FROM A SINGLE STRIKING ACCENT

TO AN ALL-OVER NEON EXPLOSION. SOME OF

THE LOOKS IN THE PAGES THAT FOLLOW INVOLVE

MULTILAYERED EFFECTS, WHILE OTHERS ADD JUST A

LITTLE SOMETHING EXTRA TO A STUNNING STAND-

ALONE COLOR. SOMETHING AS SIMPLE AS A TONE-

ON-TONE ROOT MELT OR A FLASH OF RAINBOW

FEATHERS WILL TAKE YOUR COLOR FROM SIMPLE TO

SIMPLY AMAZING. AS I'VE DISCUSSED THROUGHOUT

THIS BOOK, THESE EFFECTS CAN BE DIALED UP OR

DOWN DEPENDING ON YOUR PERSONAL STYLE.

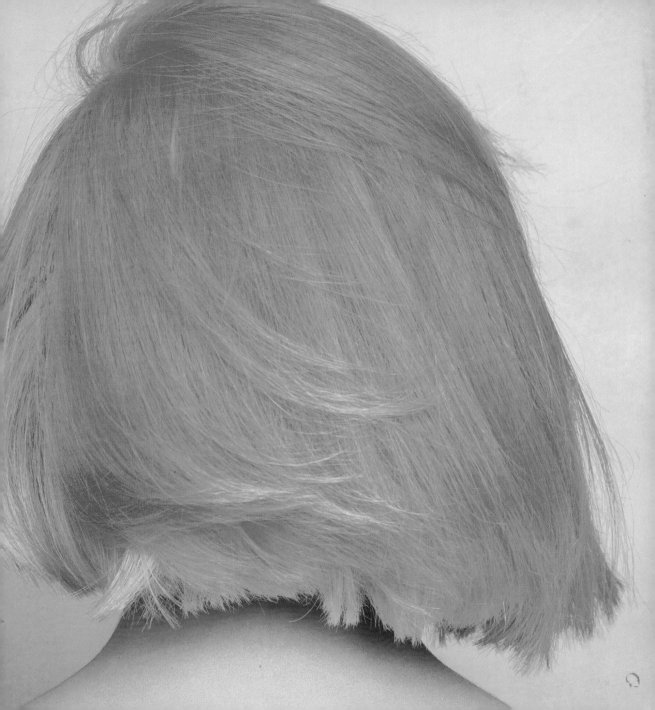

Pro Tip

This kind of tone-on-tone color melting is a great way to add depth and dimensionality to what's essentially an all-over color. Many of us rocked the "I just dumped this whole bottle of color on my head" look at some point in our teenage years. This look shows why a little extra effort has a major payoff in terms of taking your color to the next level.

NEGATIVE SPACE SHINE LINE

ROOTED NEON GREEN SHADOW MELT

This is a super fun and easy look that lets you achieve bright colors with a really nice dimension to them, courtesy of the negative space up above. You can adjust this look to use different color families if neon green isn't to your taste, or follow as is for some radioactively brilliant hair!

PREPARING THE CANVAS

Since we were using some warmer, lighter greens as part of this look, we wanted to keep Rhinny's hair a warm (but still very light!) shade. This is especially true because we were putting deeper greens next to those light ones, and deeper colors get more support from warmer tones.

We used 20 volume lightener on Rhinny's hair to bring her canvas up to a Level 9, which is ideal for showcasing the bright shades in this dye job because Level 9 hair still retains a warmth generally lacking in a Level 10.

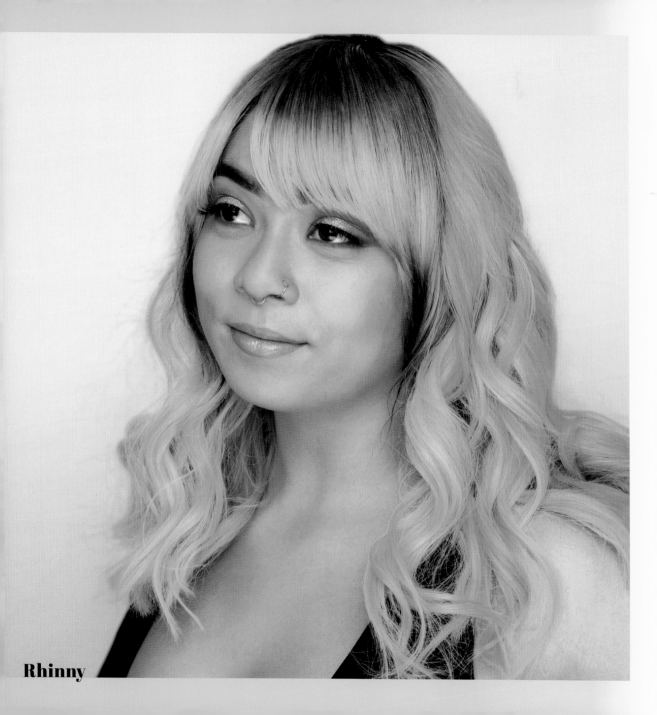

Rhinny

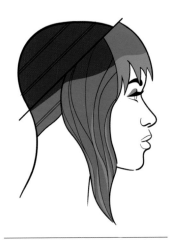

COLOR FORMULA

Root Formula

2 parts Neon Green + 1 part
Dark Green

Melting Formulas

Medium Green: 1 part Neon
Green + 1 part Bold Yellow +
¼ part Dark Green

Light Green: 1 part white
conditioner + 1 part Bold
Yellow + 1 part Electric Green

APPLYING THE COLOR

1 Decide where you want the lightest part of the fringe to be—
if you have bangs, it should be in the front of them—and
section that area of hair horizontally.

2 Apply the Root Formula to the roots of the fringe area, going
three inches down the shaft of the hair.

3 Next, take the Light Green and apply it to your fringe from
the ends up.

4 Melt the Light Green directly into the Root Formula for a
bold pop. (Do this only in the fringe!)

5 After completing the fringe, apply the root formula to the
rest of your head, going in horizontal sections and working
your way through the rest of your scalp.

6 Freehand paint on the Medium Green, with occasional
streaks of Light Green, all the way to the ends. Melt the root
formula into the main color with a clean dye brush or a fine-
tooth comb.

PROCESSING

Let process at room temperature for 30 minutes and rinse with
cold water until the water runs clear.

Since you'll end up with dark roots and very vibrant ends, hold
the ends off to the side while rinsing, so that the deeper color
won't run into the brighter ones. Once you've thoroughly rinsed
the darker areas, you should wash the ends separately.

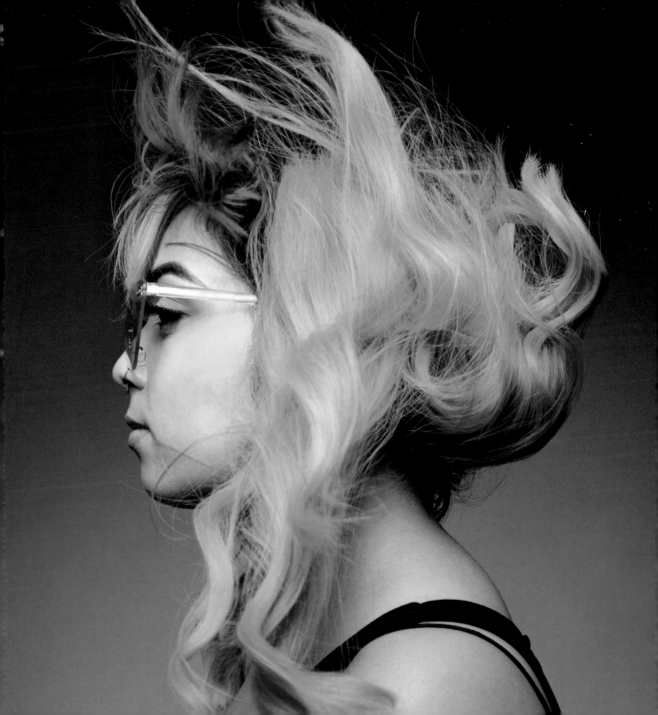

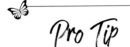

Pro Tip

When working with hair feathers,
you want to create small horizontal
shine lines that alternate and vary
in color, so that they contrast with
each other nicely. For this look,
we used light next to dark. You can
also place all-over color around
the hair feathers to showcase
them even more.

HAIR FEATHERS

This technique uses very small horizontal shine lines, in a riff on
the look created by the striped feather extensions you can clip
into your hair. Dyed hair feathers make for a really fun interplay
of color, whether you use shades that are close to each other,
direct opposites, or a neon and a black for heightened drama.
You can have a lot of fun with the placement of your section
of hair feathers, too. Have fun and use these hints to let you
customize them to be all your own.

PREPARING THE CANVAS

Madison's hair had previously been lightened, with about 2
inches of her natural root grown out. We decided to lighten her
natural root to match her Level 9 hair, leaving us with a perfectly
even canvas to work with.

APPLYING THE COLOR

1   Decide where you want your hair feathers to fall, keeping
    in mind that each hair feather should consist of a horizontal
    section about 1 inch tall and 2 inches long. Note that here,
    the hair feather is a thin layer resting on top of the pink.

2   Secure your hair feather sections out of the way with clips.
    In this case, we worked around our model's temples in a
    diagonal back placement, and mirrored that on both sides.

3   Now apply the All-Over Pink Formula to the rest of your hair,
    except for the clipped sections.

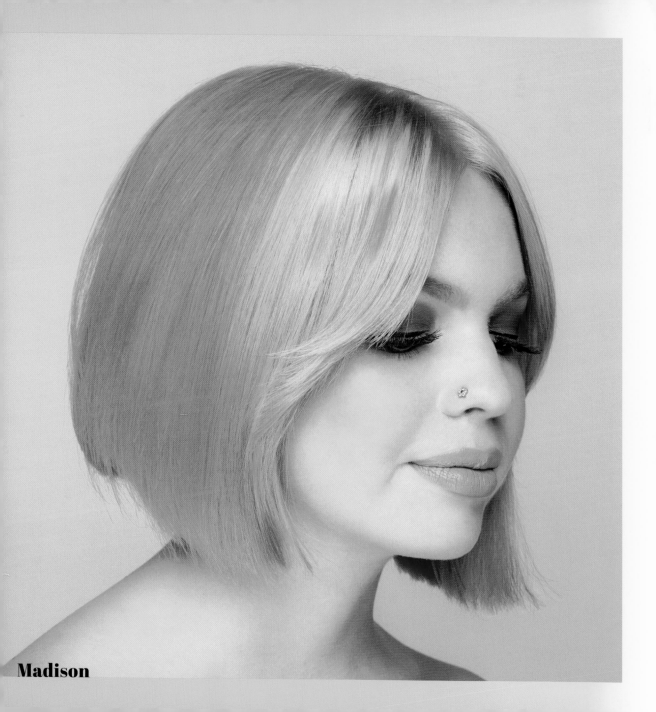

Madison

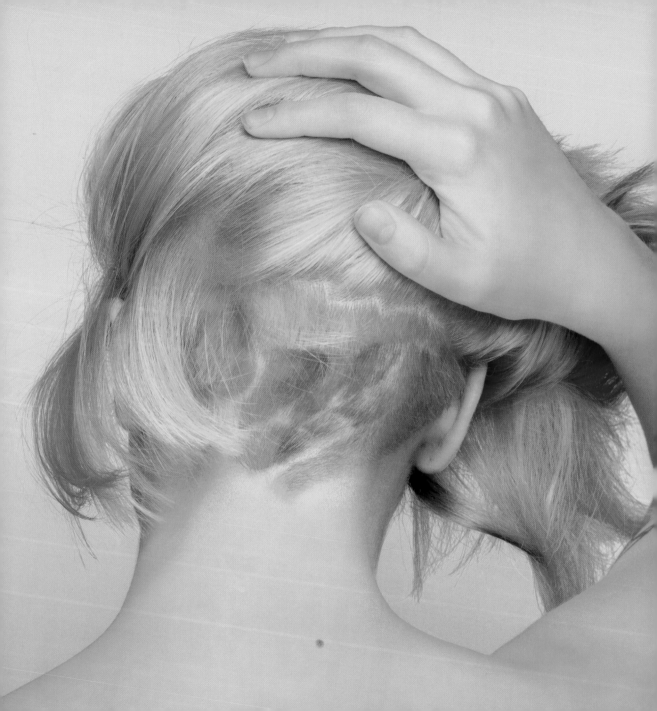

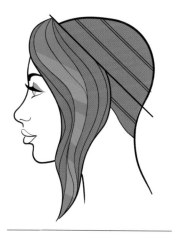

COLOR FORMULA
All-Over Pink Formula
1 part Soft Pink + 1 part
Medium Pink + 1 part
Neon Pink

Hair Feather Formulas
Mint

Neon Green

Pale Blue

4 To create the shine-line effect for your hair feathers, take your selected section of hair down from one of the clips.

5 Take the newly unclipped section of hair and place a piece of foil directly underneath to keep the color from transferring. Using the foil helps you anchor the hair while you paint and keeps the color exactly where you want it.

6 Start applying the Mint Green to the first 1 inch of your hair, starting at the roots.

7 Apply Neon Green to the next 1 inch of your hair, blending the two colors together where they meet—but keep it subtle! You want clean transitions between shine lines, not a full-on gradient.

8 Apply Pale Blue to the next 1 inch of your hair, blending it in to the color above it.

9 Continue alternating like this until you reach the end of your first section.

10 Repeat steps 4 through 9 for any other hair feathers. Note that a lot of haircuts and textures will get the tapering shown in the photo naturally, either due to layers, or because your hair thins out as it gets longer.

PROCESSING
Let process at room temperature for 30 minutes, then rinse with cold water until the water runs clear.

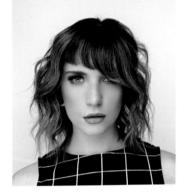

Rebecca's natural roots are a Level 5 (see the color chart on page 18).

Pro Tip

The best way to maintain unnaturally colored hair dye is to use professional, color-safe shampoos and conditioners. Limit how often you wash your hair, as the color fades with every wash. Also, wash in cold water if possible: Cold water closes down the hair shaft, reducing the amount of color that slips out. The warmer and hotter the water, the faster your color will fade.

TWO-TONE NEON SPLIT

HALF AND HALF

This is a fun technique that's not only super easy, but totally customizable. For this look, we worked with two beautiful, bold neon colors to bring this two-tone transformation to life, but really you can try it with any two complementary colors of your choice. (Check out the color wheel on page 16 for inspiration and mix it up to your heart's content.)

PREPARING THE CANVAS

Rebecca had a previous balayage, but we knew that in order to have our neons perform as brightly as we wanted, we would need to lighten her hair some more.

Rebecca has a natural Level 5 root. We decided to do finely woven highlights in order to break up her roots, and so that we could lift to Levels 8/9, utilizing the yellow undertone and working to help brighten up our formulas.

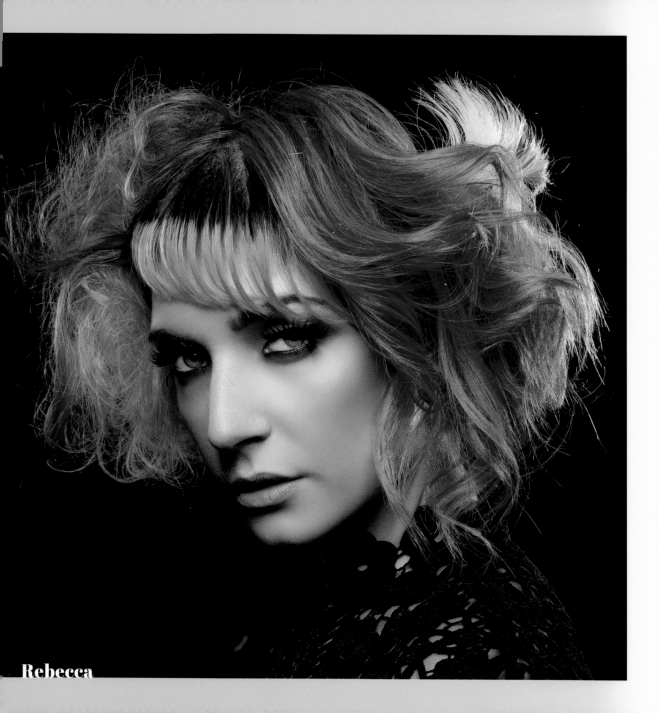

Rebecca

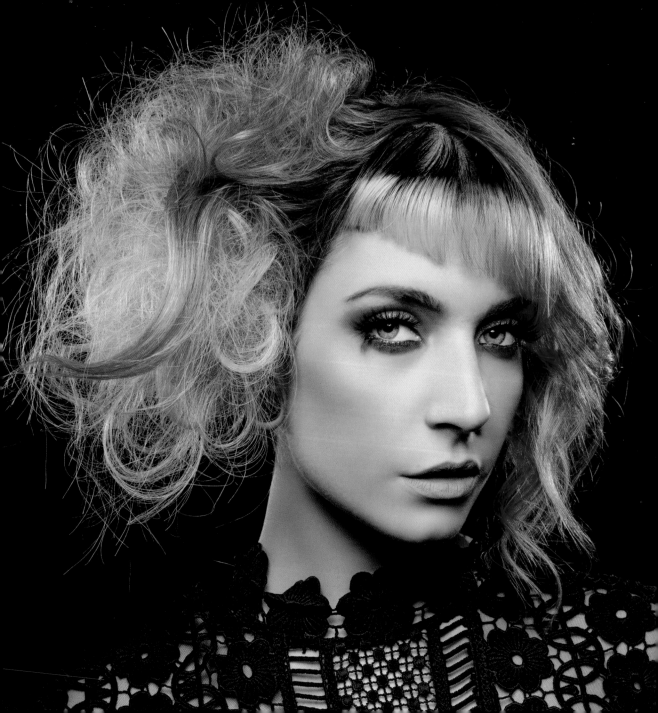

COLOR FORMULA

Neon Orange: 1 part Neon Orange + 1 part Bold Yellow

Neon Pink: 1 part Neon Pink + 1 part Soft Pink

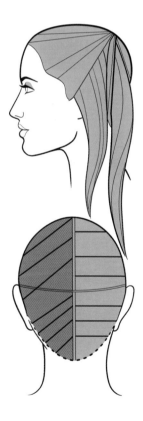

APPLYING THE COLOR

1 Decide which side you would like to start on—there's no right or wrong (just right and left!).

2 On that side, split the hair into horizontal sections and begin applying the color, softly blending the sections together from roots to ends.

3 Repeat Step 2 with the other half of the head, using the opposite color formula.

PROCESSING

Let your color process at room temperature for 30 minutes and rinse with cold water until the water runs clear.

Jordyn's natural hair is a Level 5/6 (see the color chart on page 18).

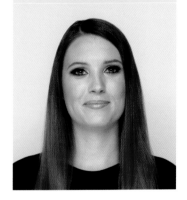

Pro Tips

If you're applying cooler colors next to warmer colors, rinsing in cold water is vital. Using warm or hot water will cause the dye to run, potentially muddling the colors.

Anytime you're working with a darker root, you will want to rinse the roots first and the rest of the hair second, so that you don't have to worry about your ends soaking up the other colors. Otherwise, you risk leaving your end color dull or muted.

SIMPLE COLOR MELT/OMBRE

ETERNAL FLAME

This beautiful color melt gets us all fired up! If you're looking to spice up your style, then this transformation is for you. This horizontal melt will be easy to blend from roots to ends, but in order to keep the vibrancy of your orange and not allow your red to overpower it, you'll want to take a few careful steps to achieve this fiery effect.

PREPARING THE CANVAS

Jordyn started off with a medium-brown canvas—in other words, a Level 5/6 warm brown. Since we knew we would be utilizing warmer reds and oranges—which show up better over browns and yellows than cold colors do—we only needed to lift our canvas up to Level 8.

We used lightener to bring up her overall hair color, but we didn't apply it to her roots, because one of our goals was to maintain a natural root that we could apply a demipermanent dye to in our second step, with a plan to continue melting our fire formulas from that section of hair.

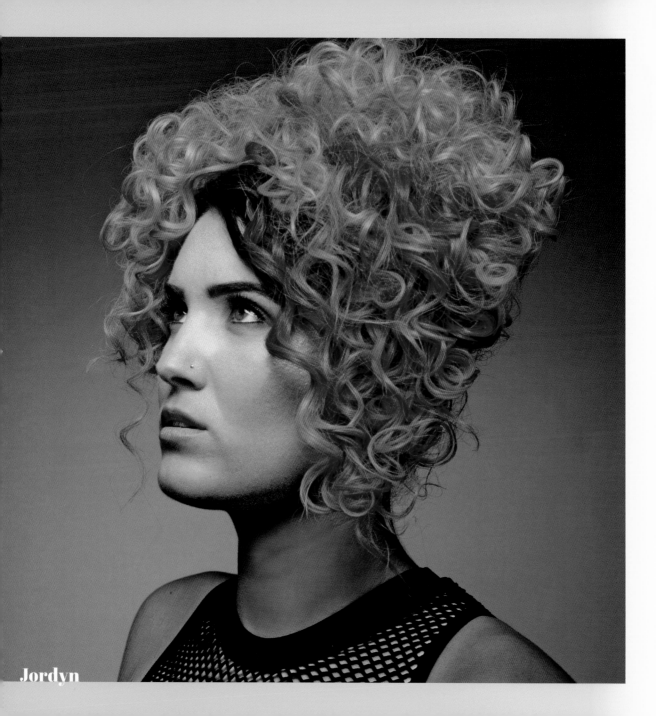
Jordyn

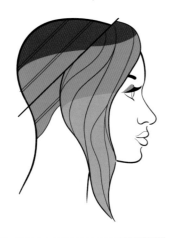

COLOR FORMULA

Root Formula
(demipermanent colors)

2 parts Bold Red +
2 parts Deep Red +
1 part Deep Violet

Midshaft Formula
Bold Red

End Formula
2 parts Neon Orange +
1 part Bold Red +
1 part Bold Yellow

APPLYING THE COLOR

1 Apply the plum-toned Root Formula to damp hair. We used a demipermanent color here to create a deep, long-lasting root that will serve as foundation for the creative color overlays to come.

2 Divide the hair into horizontal sections.

3 Apply the Root Formula, moving horizontally around your head and working the dye the into the first 3 inches of your hair.

4 Let the Root Formula process for 25 minutes.

5 Rinse out your roots and blow-dry.

6 Next, resection the hair and apply the Midshaft Formula to the next 3 inches of your hair, feathering and melting it into the root section as you go.

7 For the last and brightest color, start at the tips of your hair and work back up toward the midshaft area. This will ensure that you're not dragging your reds into your orange, which is important, because if the colors blend together too much, you'll lose the striking differentiation you see here.

PROCESSING

Let process for 30 minutes at room temperature. Rinse in cold water in two stages: first, rinse only the midshaft, holding your hair up by the ends to protect them (to the best of your ability-- it's not always possible to do this precisely, especially without an extra pair of hands to help!). Finally, rinse your ends.

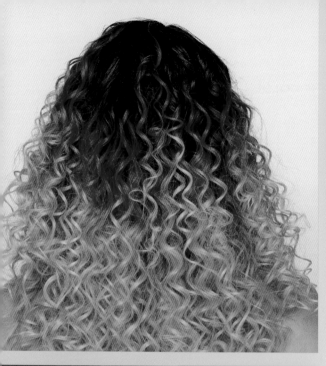
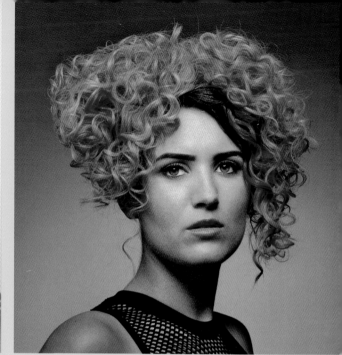
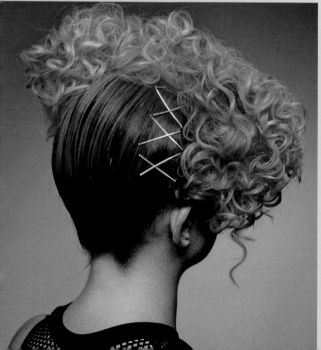
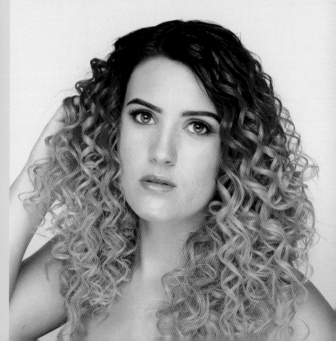

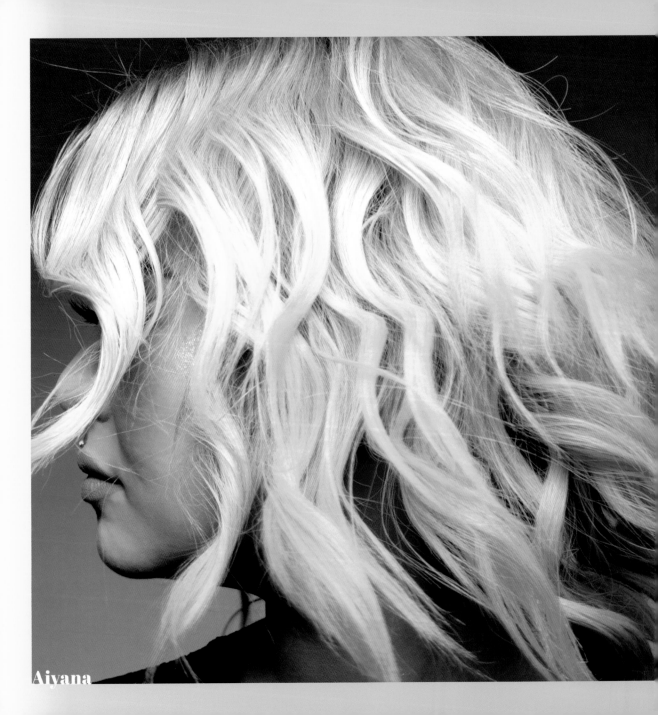

Aiyana

COLOR MELT
DIPPED TIPS

This versatile look provides a pop of color for a couple different techniques, whether you're creating a truly vibrant spectacle or giving a little edge to your corporate look.

Dipped tips can be a great pop for an ombre, freshening up an existing look, or you can recreate what we have done on our model here by fully lightening your hair and then applying a bright yellow tip dip. (Sadly, this look doesn't actually involve dipping your hair into a giant vat of dye. The rhyming name was just too hard to resist.)

PREPARING THE CANVAS
For this transformation, we lightened Aiyana up to a high Level 9. After the lightening was done, we toned her hair using white conditioner mixed with a bit of light silver and soft purple semipermanent dye. That sort of mixture is a really nice, cheap trick you can use when you don't want to buy a separate toner. We let the toner process for 10 minutes, then shampooed and completely blow-dried her hair before applying the dye.

Pro Tip

When you have bold tips that are melting into another color up above them, it can help to start by applying dye to the higher sections of the hair first. Once the root and midshaft dye is on, start down at the very ends of your hair, and work up toward the other colors. Doing that will help keep the ends as light and bright as possible, so that the other colors don't melt downward into the ends and cause the focus or vibrancy of tip color to be lost.

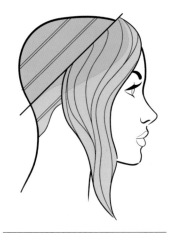

COLOR FORMULA

Root Formula
1 part white conditioner +
1 part Light Silver + 1 part
Soft Purple + 1 part
Soft Pink + 1 part Mint

End Formula
1 part white conditioner +
1 part Bold Yellow

APPLYING THE COLOR

1 Section your hair horizontally.

2 Apply your Root Formula throughout the hair in the horizontal sections you made, working all the way around your head. Apply it as far down as you want the color to go. For our look, we did about half of Aiyana's hair.

3 For a more choppy and dimensional look, vary how far down the root color goes by an inch or two on random sections.

4 Once you're done applying the first formula, take your End Formula and start applying it to the very tips of your hair.

5 Work from the tips of the hair upward, melting and blending the color into the root formula.

PROCESSING

Process the hair at room temperature for 30 minutes and rinse with cold water until the water runs clear.

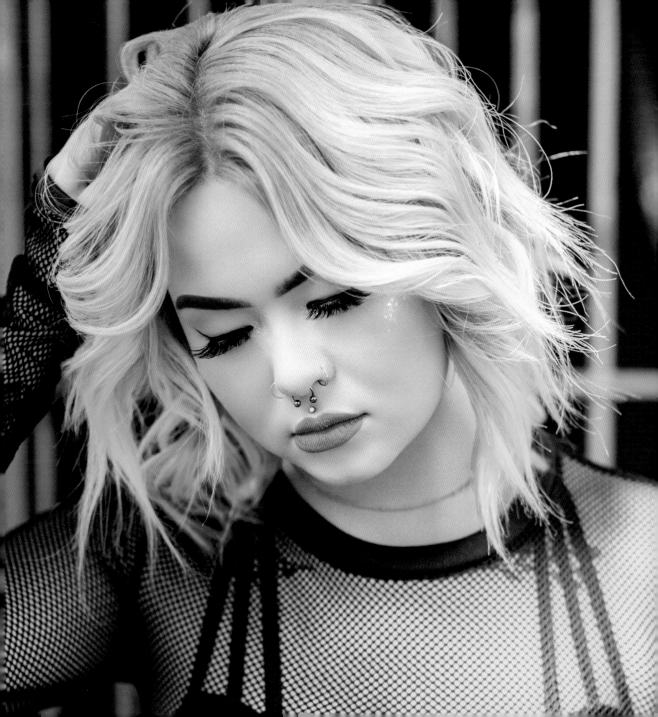

Megan's natural roots are a Level 5 (see the color chart on page 18).

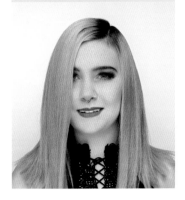

Pro Tip

If you have an existing creative color that you want or need to remove before trying out a new look, don't just go for bleaching it out. This can be damaging to the hair and, maybe even worse, chemical interactions can leave you with some unexpected tones. Instead, use a gentle color remover specially formulated for semipermanent dyes.

MODIFIED COLOR MELT

LASER ROOTS

This colorful technique is all about creating a brighter focus on the root of the hair. Neon formulations can be great for these looks. For Megan's hair we went with a neon yellow, but this technique is very versatile and can be created using any neon formulation you like.

Once you've gotten a chance to play you will see the options are endless and you have the freedom to be the artist. And don't just play with color—go crazy with the style too, crazy enough to match the zany dye.

PREPARING THE CANVAS

To achieve this vibrant color, we had to lift Megan's Level 5 roots about 4 levels, to a Level 8 or 9, before doing anything else. Because the final effect uses a yellow, the aim was to lift to a yellowish tone that would best support that dye. We then used a color remover to take out the leftover green she had from a previous dye job.

If you're prepping your hair at home, you can often wash out a lot of an old semipermanent color by doing the opposite of what we recommend in most cases! Wash your hair frequently in hot water, as hot as you can stand, using clarifying shampoo. This won't necessarily remove all of your old color, but it will fade it considerably.

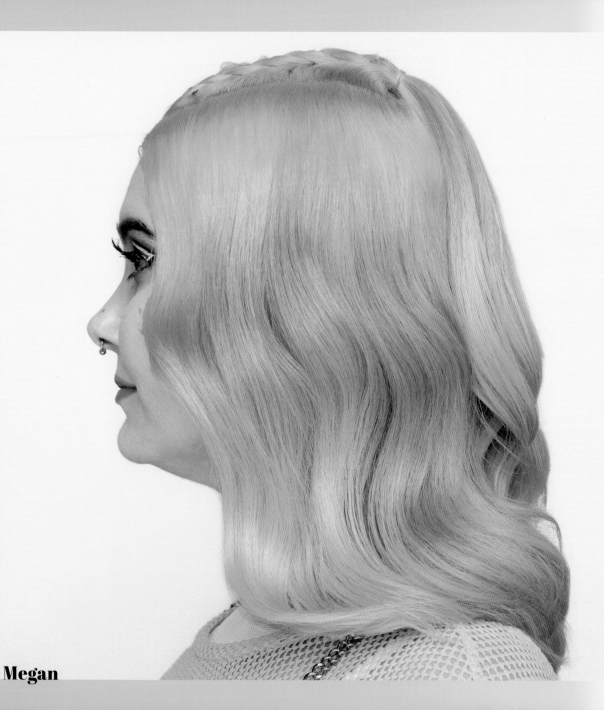

Megan

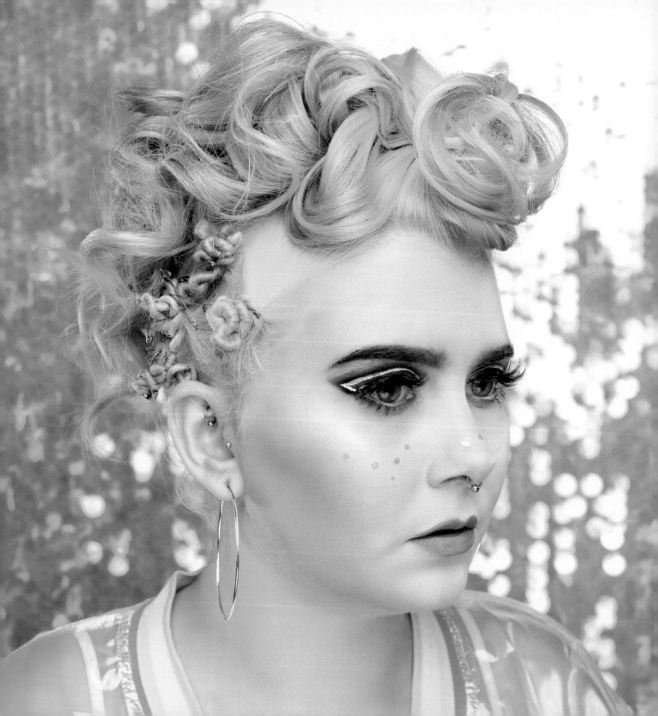

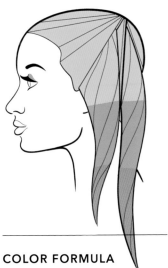

COLOR FORMULA
Root Formula
Bold Yellow

Midshaft Formula
1 part white conditioner +
1 part Mint + 1 part Pastel Blue

End Formula
1 part white conditioner +
1 part Neon Orange

APPLYING THE COLOR

1 Determine how many inches you would like your laser root to be. This is all personal preference.

2 Start applying your root formula at the scalp, brushing downward.

3 After you have applied your Root Formula, hold each section with light tension at a zero degree elevation, which means straight down, and start to apply your midshaft formula.

4 Softly feather and blend the formulas together where they meet, and then pull the dye brush down further to melt down the hair shaft.

5 Now, for the ends. We went with a subtle pop on the ends, so we only applied the End Formula to the last 2 inches of each section. A great way to do this is to save the ends for last, then just hold the ends horizontally, using your hand as a guide for how high to apply the formula. Follow that around the head until all of the ends are evenly saturated.

PROCESSING
Allow your color to process at room temperature for 30 minutes. Rinse with cold water only, and do not shampoo afterwards, so that your colors don't bleed together.

Semipermanent colors are conditioning to the hair so you don't need to condition. To ensure all of the color is rinsed out you want to keep rinsing until the water runs clear.

Pro Tip

For this color technique, both placement and balance are key. Consider not only your hair cut's shape but the shape of your head itself to help you decide how you want your halos and how to personalize them.

COLOR FADING

NEON URBAN HALO FADE

We created this look with Jordan's texture and haircut in mind. It's the different shades in the same color family—going from a darker outer ring to a lighter inner ring—that make this transformation so eye-catching.

After you apply this dye job, and are out in the world, be sure to make at least 113 jokes about how impressive your halo is and what an absolute angel you are.

PREPARING THE CANVAS

Jordan had his natural Level 3 hair previously lifted to a high Level 9. Because of that, we were able to utilize his preexisting blonde canvas for our blue color palette.

We decided to not tone Jordan before to applying his colors—but if your canvas has too much underlying yellow pigment, I suggest neutralizing the warmth so that your blue formulas will be true to tone. If there's too much of a yellow undertone, your blues will come out teal.

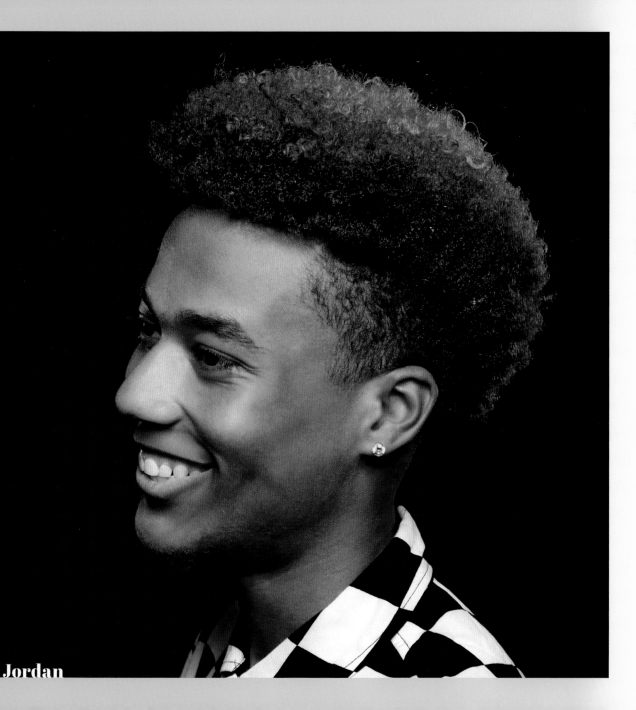

Jordan

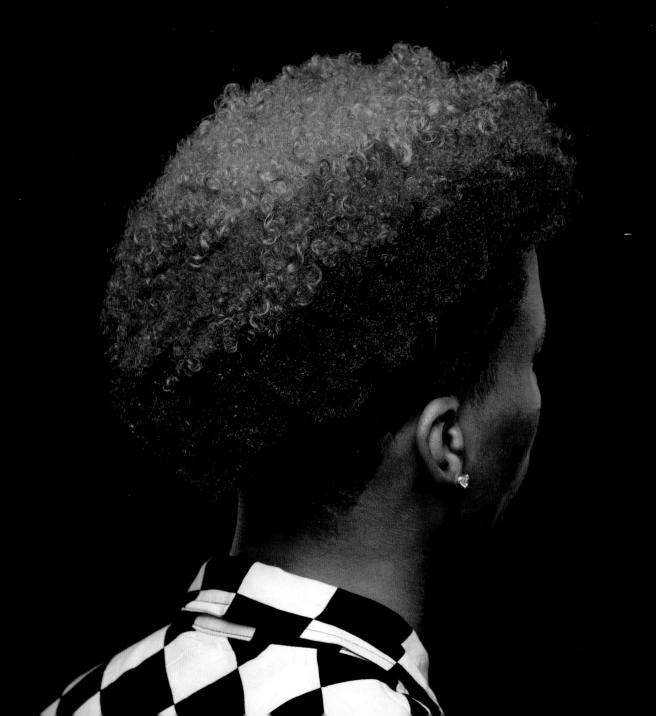

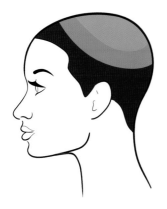

COLOR FORMULA
Outer Halo Formula
Deep Blue

Middle Halo Formula
2 parts Medium Vibrant Blue +
1 part Deep Blue

Inner Halo Formula
2 parts Medium Vibrant Blue +
1 part Pastel Blue

APPLYING THE COLOR

1 First, figure out where you want your halos to go.

2 Start adding color in the outer halo, which should be
   the darkest formula. With kinky, curly hair like Jordan's,
   it's important to take one small section at a time and be
   sure to fully saturate each one.

3 Start by working on one the side of your head. Move
   around to the temples, then fringe, and continue to
   follow the section around the head, making sure to have your
   halo fully saturated and balanced—the same size
   and width all around.

4 Next, begin to apply the medium color to the area you
   picked as your middle halo, working right next to your outer
   halo. Repeat Step 2, working around your head until your
   second halo is fully saturated.

5 Your last, inner halo will be your lightest formula, and it'll
   bring a great focal point, so make sure that you plan and
   double-check that your plan for this inner ring is nicely
   balanced before beginning.

6 Take small sections, and make sure to saturate all of your hair
   evenly and completely.

PROCESSING
Let process at room temperature for 30 minutes and rinse with
cold water until the water runs clear.

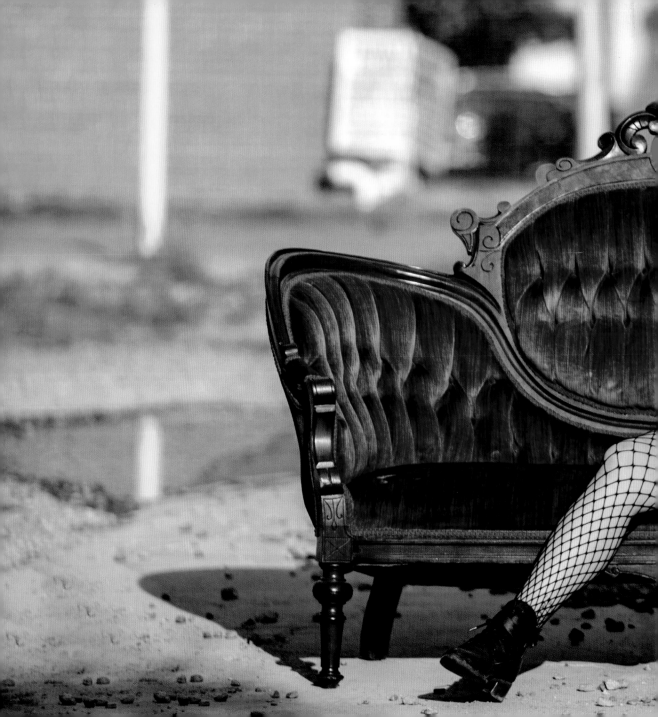

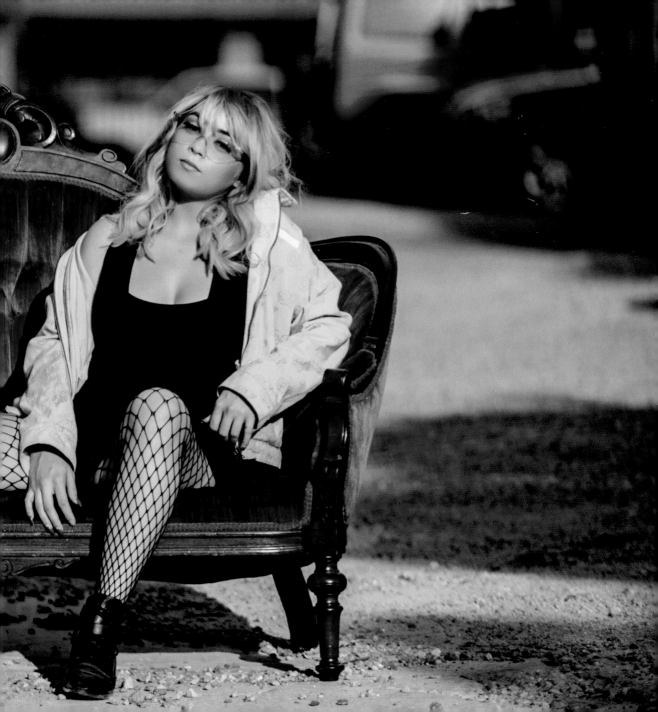

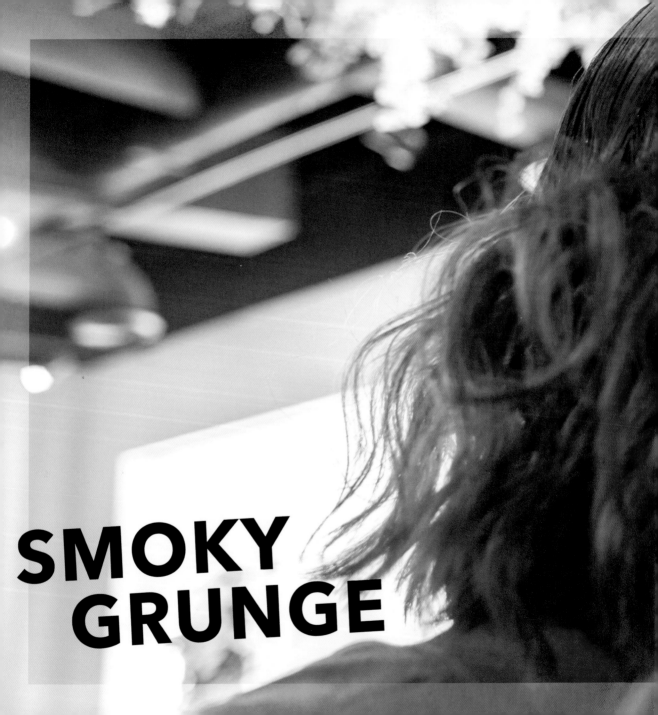

SMOKY GRUNGE

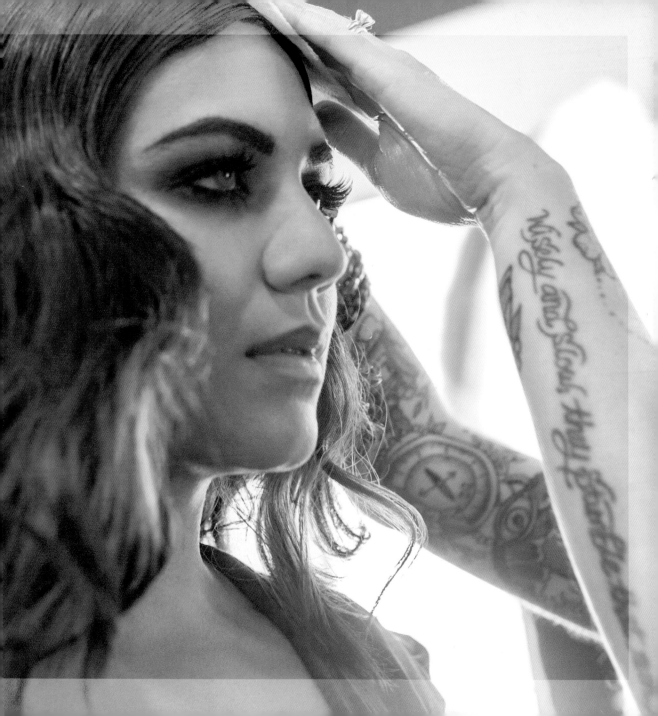

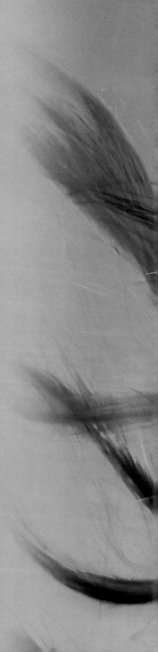

Where There's Smoke

THE LOOKS IN THIS CHAPTER ARE INSPIRED BY

THE GRUNGE MUSIC AND FASHION TRENDS

OF THE 80S AND 90S—A LITTLE DOWNBEAT, A

LITTLE PUNK, A LITTLE STREET, AND DEFINITELY

NOT NEON OR PASTEL. THEY RANGE FROM

UNDERSTATED LOOKS THAT CAN GO FROM

THE OFFICE TO A DIVE BAR WITH EASE TO AN

ABSOLUTELY GORGEOUS GOTH-INSPIRED DARK

MERMAID EFFECT. WHETHER YOU'RE LOOKING

TO TRY SOMETHING A LITTLE UNUSUAL, OR ON

A QUEST FOR THE PERFECT COLOR TO BRING

OUT YOUR SULTRY SIDE, THESE SMOLDERING

STYLES WILL FIT THE BILL.

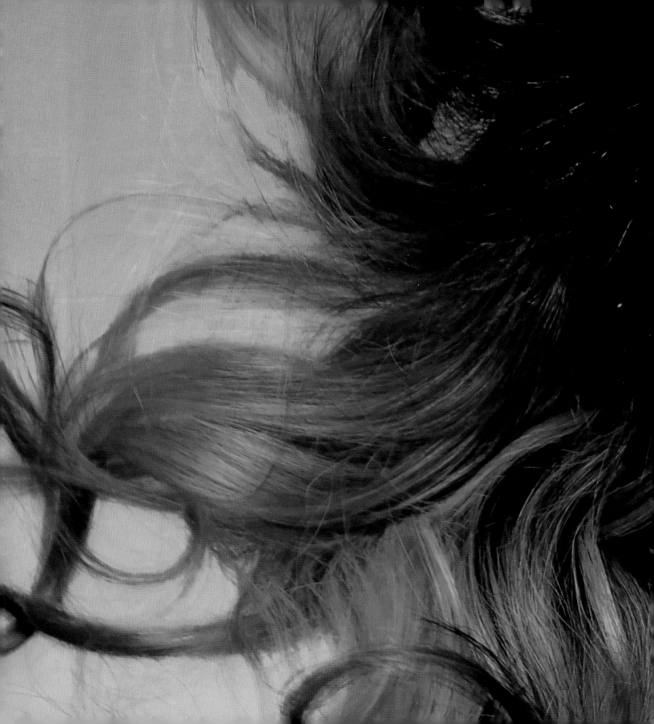

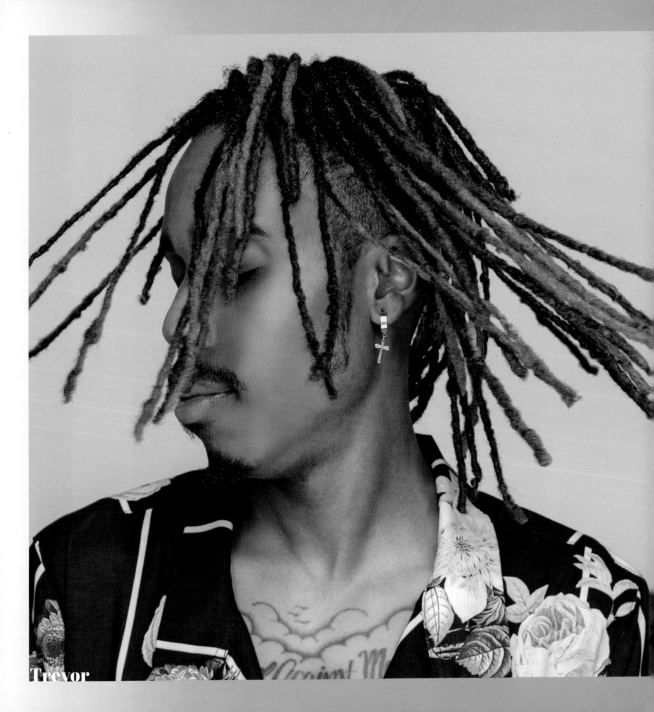

Trevor

COLOR MELT

GREEN GRUNGE DREAD MELT

We transformed Trevor's awesome dreadlocks with a grungy green melt, allowing different dimensions of green to blend into and around each other. This is a great way to create really cool variation and dimension that flows naturally with your hair and its movement.

PREPARING THE CANVAS

Trevor's hair had previously been lifted and colored blue. The blue had faded quite a bit, but we decided it would be best to lift out all the remaining color and start with a fresh canvas. When working with dreads and lightener, a few things are key: First, make sure the hair is human before applying lightener, and that the hair itself are in good shape. Given how tightly dread are wrapped, it's important to make sure you're fully saturating each one.

We let our lightener process for 40 minutes. After rinsing, we discovered that the blue had not been lifted out as much as we hoped. It had shifted to a green, but it still lacked the lightness we were going for. We didn't want to risk damaging Trevor's hair, so instead of lightening it further, we followed up with two clarifying shampoo rinses, working each dreadlock in our hands, in order to remove the residual color from of the hair. That left us with a canvas that worked perfectly for a nice, grungy green.

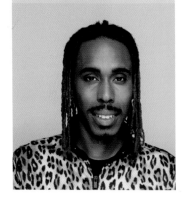

Trevor's natural roots are a Level 1/2 (see the color chart on page 18).

Pro Tip

Trevor's natural hair color didn't have a lot of underlying warmth to it, and we wanted to warm him up for this effect. If you've got a similar canvas, whether it's your natural color or the result of previous dye jobs, you can correct for that by adding a bit of a warmer tone to your color formula. Here, a jolt of yellow in the green base color did the trick.

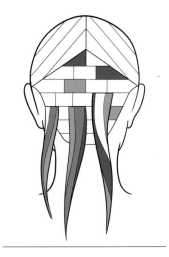

COLOR FORMULA

Dark Green: 1 part Deep Green + 1 part Deep Teal

Medium Green: 1 part Deep Green + 1 part Bold Yellow

Light Green: 1 part Bold Yellow + 1 part Electric Green + 1 part Deep Green

APPLYING THE COLOR

1   Pick one side of the front of your head to start with.

2   Apply the three colors as desired in a bricklay fashion—meaning the different patches of color are offset from each other, from dread to dread, and the borders between colors don't line up, as in a brick wall.

3   Try to apply the lightest shade of green to the areas where the hair is the lightest, and work from there. Doing that will let you benefit from the underlying warmth of the hair and get brighter accents for your end result.

4   Keep going until the desired areas of hair are completely covered, melting the colors into each other as desired.

PROCESSING

Let process at room temperature for 30 minutes and rinse with cold water until the water runs clear.

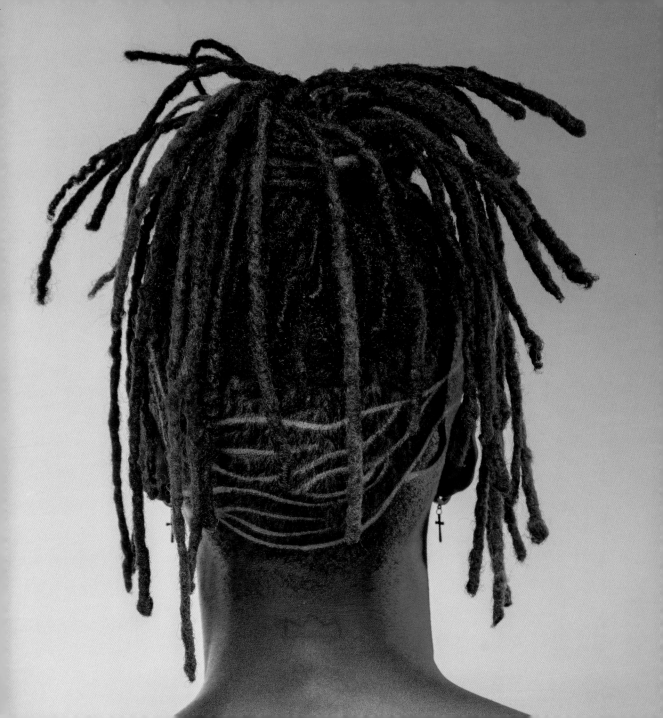

Jenny's natural hair is a Level 2 (see the color chart on page 18).

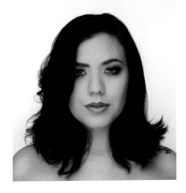

Pro Tip

A really good way to help keep your shine lines controlled and your painting precise is to use clear meche sheets. These prefab strips help you keep your sections divided, like foils do—but unlike foils, they're see through, so they can give you some really useful visual guidance as you work. Hold the hair directly on the meche as you paint on your colors; the dye will make it stick.

SHINE LINES

DARK RAINBOW

This look is great for people with darker hair because it doesn't require lightening the hair nearly as far as the bright and pastel looks do. It's also perfect for adding a subtler accent to any hair.

Shine lines are a brilliant optical illusion that make it look like a rainbow laser beam has been projected onto your head. Traditionally, they're done by applying bright hues to the hair in horizontal, diagonal, or overlapping lines. We're keeping the traditional shape for this one, but when it comes to the color? We're gonna be rebels.

PREPARING THE CANVAS

Jenny has very dark natural hair, so we knew that lifting it would be a challenge. That's why we went with a more muted shine line—dark colors and warm dyes don't require you to lighten your hair as much. That's a huge asset in this case, one that let us create this exquisite, dark, and almost gothic look.

Given her natural Level 2 hair color, we lightened a wide horizontal strip of her hair up to a Level 6/7, but left the top 4 and bottom 3 inches darker. Another benefit to the warm colors used is that we didn't have to tone her hair.

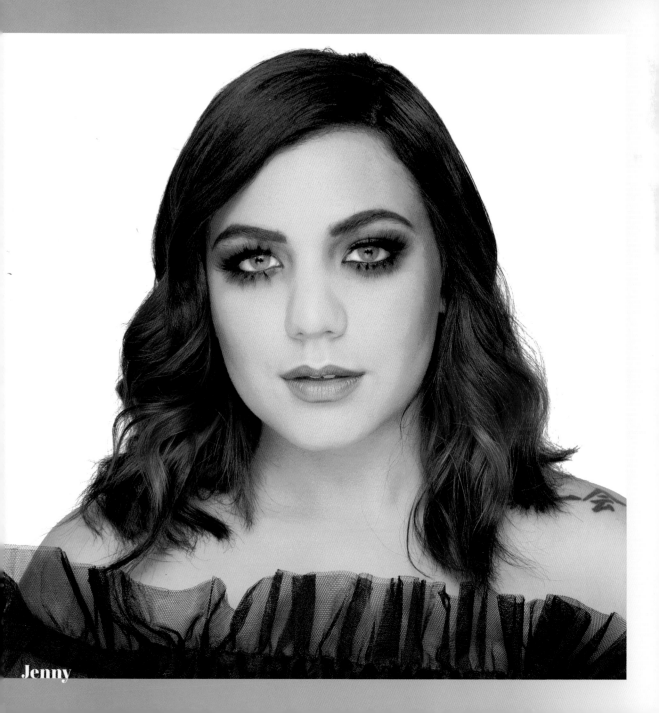

Jenny

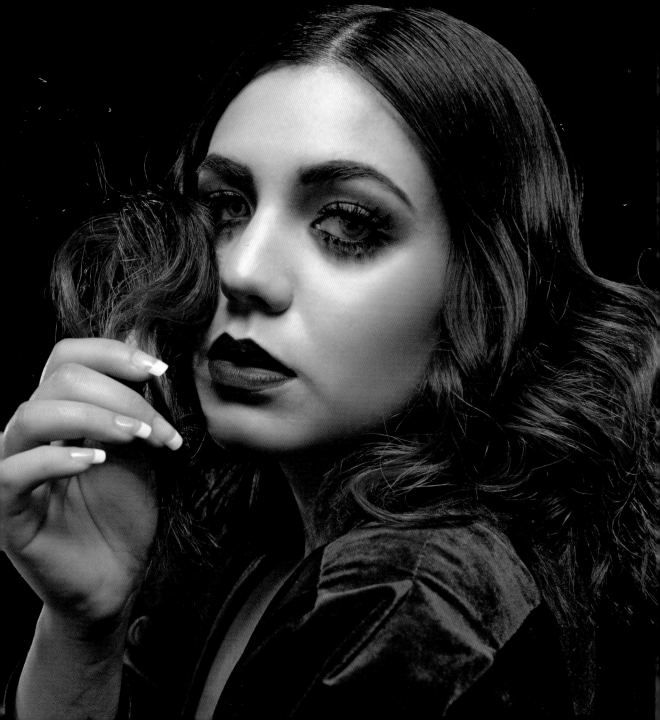

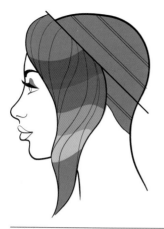

COLOR FORMULA
Root and End Formula
1 part Deep Blue +
1 part Medium Vibrant Blue

Shine Line Formulas
Purple: 1 part Deep Violet +
1 part Fuchsia

Red: 1 part Bold Red +
1 part Deep Red

Orange: 1 part Bold Red +
1 part Neon Orange +
1 part Bold Yellow

Yellow: Bold Yellow

APPLYING THE COLOR

1 Starting at the nape of your neck, take a 1-inch section of hair, hold it straight down, and put a meche or foil sheet underneath it. Now apply the Root Formula to the first 2 inches of this section.

2 On the same section of hair, apply 2 inches of Purple, starting at the bottom edge of the Root Formula. Blend the two formulas into each other for a smooth transition.

3 Apply Red to the next 2 inches of your section, then melt that transition together.

4 Apply Orange to the next 2 inches and melt together.

5 Apply Yellow to the rest of the lightened hair, ideally another 2 inches, blending as you go.

6 When you're satisfied with the color melt, wrap the meche strip around the dyed hair to prevent cross-contamination.

7 Repeat Steps 1–6, moving from the nape of your neck to the crown of your head. As you go, lay each new section over the previous, wrapped one, letting it serve as a guide. Do the same on the right and left sides of your head.

PROCESSING
Let process at room temperature for 30 minutes and rinse with cold water. Rinse the roots and ends first, holding the shine lines out of the water, so that the deeper and darker colors don't run into the brighter ends.

Meghan's pre-dyed hair was lifted to a Level 9/10 (see the color chart on page 18).

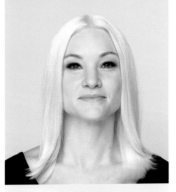

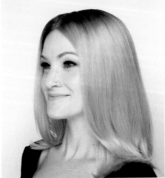

BLUE JEANS COLOR MELT

SMOKY DENIM

This color palette is a crowd-pleaser—lots of people have blue hair these days, but few of them know how to obtain a cool, smooth effect like this. We created the perfect Smoky Blue Jeans look to take your style to the next level, using a simple color melt for the perfect cool, jeans-inspired tone.

PREPARING THE CANVAS

Meghan's hair was lifted to a high Level 9/10. Since we were working with the cooler smoky blues, we decided to tone her canvas to an icy, smoky light silver before applying our color melt. For a cool shade of dye like this, it's better to tone the hair with something icy, so we mixed a semipermanent icy silver dye in white conditioner to make our DIY toner.

Pro Tip

The Neon Orange is added to the root formula in order to neutralize the blue base of the silvers and make a true slate gray.

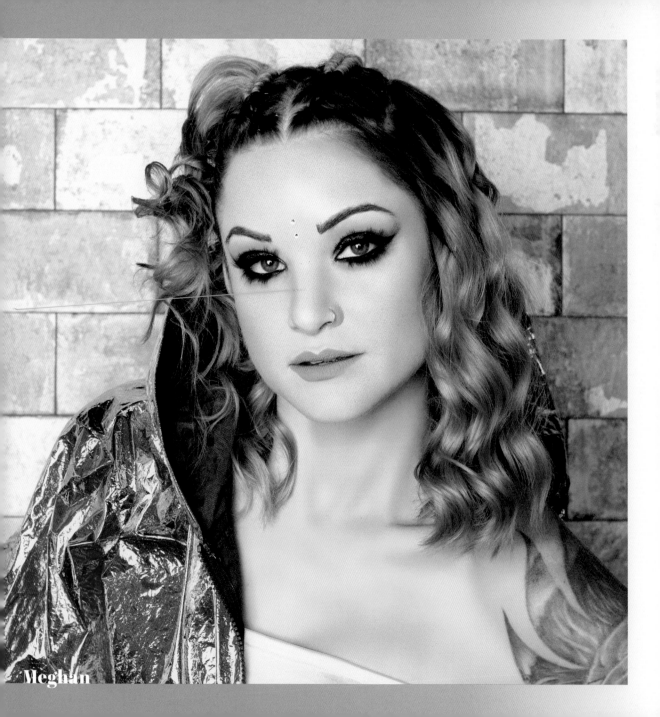
Meghan

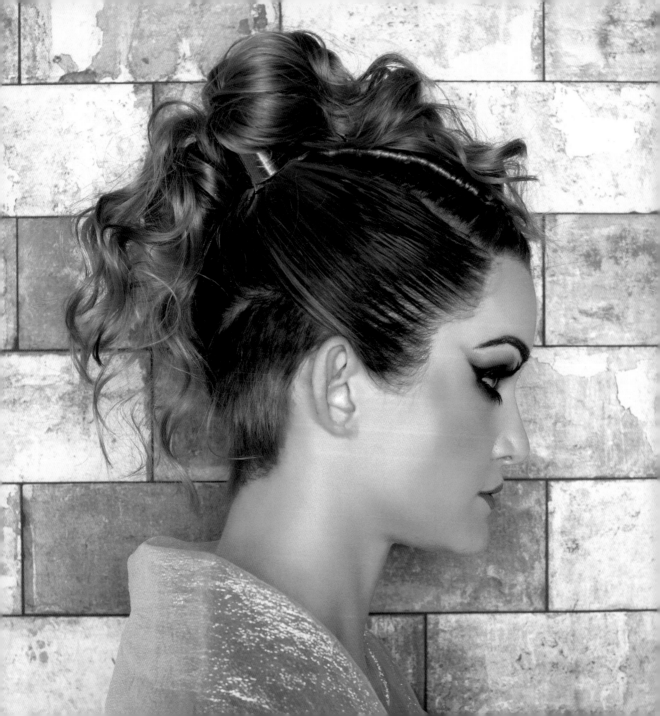

COLOR FORMULA
Root Formula
1 part Light Silver + 1 part Dark Silver + 1 part Soft Purple + 1 part Neon Orange

Main Formula
3 parts white conditioner + 3 parts Light Silver + 3 parts Pastel Blue + 1 part Medium Vibrant Blue

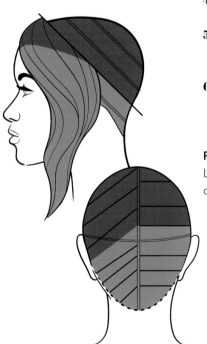

APPLYING THE COLOR

1   Section your hair off horizontally, so that all of the hair in each section starts from approximately the same height on your head.

2   Take the Root Formula and apply it to the first 1 or 2 inches of your hair, starting directly on your scalp.

3   Work the root color around the rest of your head, trying to keep the length of the dyed portion consistent as you go.

4   Section your hair horizontally again.

5   Begin applying the Main Formula from the end of your root color down to your ends.

6   As you apply the Main Formula, blend and melt it into the Root Formula by using the brush to mix them back and forth across the border.

PROCESSING
Let process at room temperature for 30 minutes and rinse with cold water until the water runs clear.

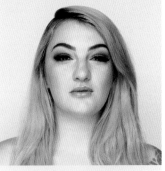

Alex's natural roots are a Level 5 (see the color chart on page 18).

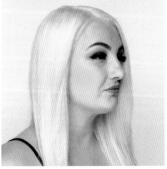

Pro Tip

To help keep your shine lines controlled and your painting precise, you'll want to use clear meche sheets.

SHINE LINE

MAGICAL MERMAID

If you love this look, now you can give yourself the rippling-in-the-water mermaid hair you've always dreamed of. Shine lines are a super fun, customizable way to make your hair stand out in the crowd. A lot of shine lines are done using bright, neon hues, but this look is bold enough it doesn't need those in-your-face hues to carry it.

PREPARING THE CANVAS

Alex had 4 inches of Level 5 hair, and the rest of her canvas was prelightened and had some old, faded teal dye left on it. In order to make sure everything came out the way we wanted, we needed to lighten her canvas to make it all a uniform color.

We started by lightening her natural root to a high Level 9. We were careful not to overlap the lightener we were applying to her roots with the faded teal section, to avoid any chemical breakage—lightening your hair too many times can do some seriously nasty stuff. Any time you're lightening hair that's been multiple colors beforehand, it's critical to take your time and do it carefully, concentrating on one color area at a time. After the more intense lightening on Alex's roots, which used 25 volume lightener, we applied a much less intense 10 volume to the ends, just to remove the faded blue.

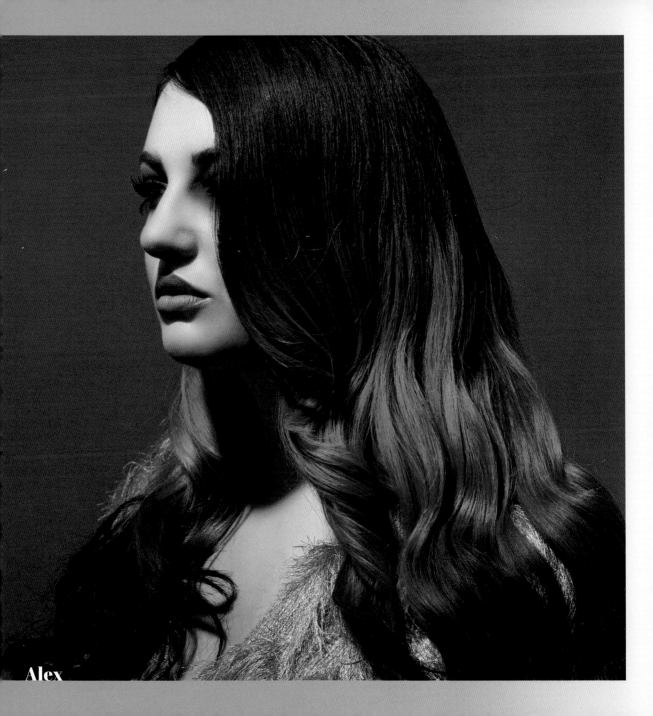

Alex

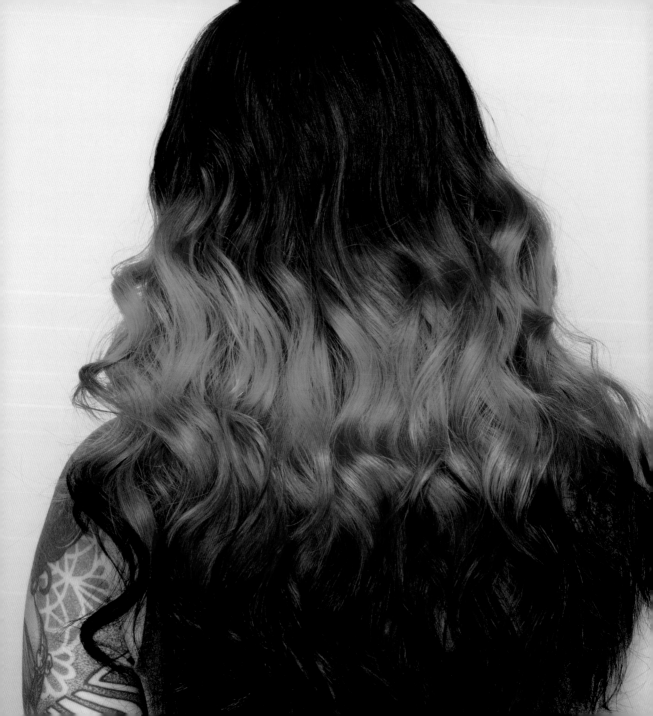

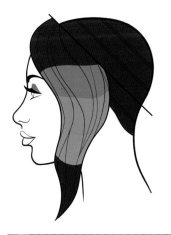

COLOR FORMULA
Root and End Formula
Midnight Blue:
3 parts Deep Blue +
1 part Black

Vibrant Blue

Bright Green

Soft Purple

APPLYING THE COLOR

1 At the nape of your neck, take a 1-inch, slightly diagonal back section, and lay it on a meche strip. Holding it straight down, paint the Root Formula on the first 6 inches of hair.

2 Apply Vibrant Blue right below the Root Formula, for the next 3 inches, melting into the root color.

3 Next, apply Bright Green to the next 3 inches of your hair, blending it into the blue as you go.

4 Apply Soft Purple to the next 3 inches; melt into Bright Green.

5 Finally, take the End Formula and apply it from the end of the shine line to the ends of your hair. Once again, melt the colors together where they meet.

6 Once you've finished your first section, wrap it in the meche strip to seal it off and keep the color from transferring.

7 Take the next section. Put a meche strip under it, and hold it on top of your first section, so that the first section can serve as a guide. Repeat up the back of your head, to the crown.

8 Repeat the same steps on both sides, continuing to layer the sections over each other so that the dye lines match.

PROCESSING
Let process at room temperature for 30 minutes and rinse with cold water. Rinse roots and ends first, holding the shine lines out of the water, so that the deeper and darker colors don't run.

NEGATIVE SPACE SHINE LINE

NEON GRUNGE LIGHT SOURCE

The idea of light sourcing comes from the field of art, and its definitions of shade, light, and form. I interpret it as highlights and contours for the hair, which are perfectly exemplified by this technique. Here, you'll be applying different colors in vertical halos, starting at the hairline and going backward. As you continue, you'll be working in deeper colors, to create a beautiful, contoured cascade.

One of my favorite ways to use this technique is to work in the same family of colors, such as light purple, into medium purple, into a dark purple at the crown of the head. The instructions here show you how to make three halos, but you can also use more, or fewer—whatever you'd like. Be creative!

PREPARING THE CANVAS

Our model Cici had already had her hair lightened, which meant we had to be careful about using more lightener, to avoid damaging her hair. This was especially true because Cici has coarse, dark hair—specifically, a natural Level 4/5—which can definitely make lifting more challenging. But her natural root was about 4 inches long, so we lightened the roots with 20 Volume lightener in order to match the rest of her hair.

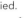

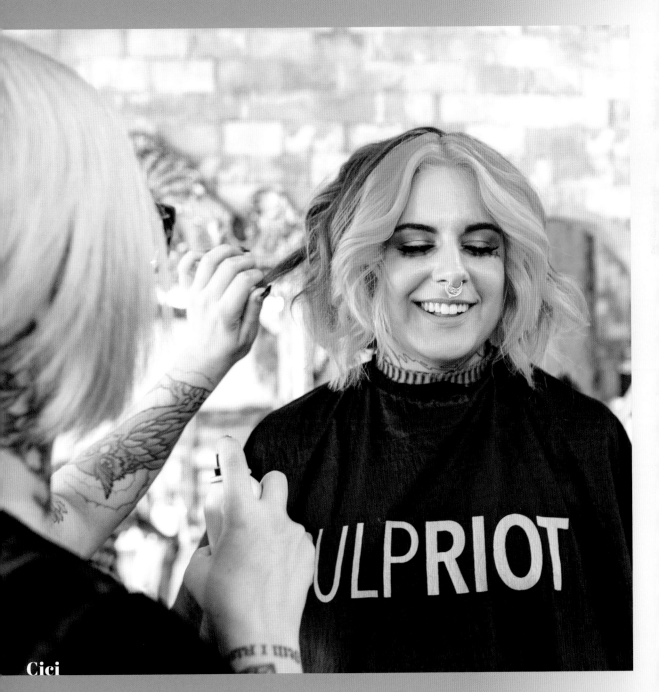

Cici

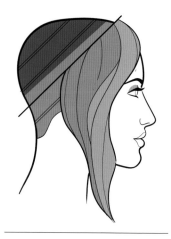

COLOR FORMULA

Zone 1 Formula

1 part white conditioner +
1 part Neon Orange + 1 part
Light Yellow + 1 part Soft Pink

Zone 2 Formula

1 part white conditioner +
1 part Neon Orange

Zone 3 Formula

1 part Light Silver + 1 part
Medium Silver + 1 part Soft
Purple + 1 part Neon Orange

APPLYING THE COLOR

1 Decide on the positioning of each halo. This technique is
one that should be customized from haircut to haircut and
person to person. For example, with shorter hair or layers,
you may want to give the crown halo—the one at the back
of the head—more width and overcompensation, so that it
brings you a beautiful veil.

2 Start in the front, with Zone 1—going front to back will make
each section easier to work with. Clip back or tie off the rest
of your hair so it stays out of your way, and then apply the
color starting at the roots and moving down to the ends.

3 Once you've completed Zone 1, if you want, you can saran
wrap the dyed hair to keep the color from transferring.

4 Move to Zone 2, the middle zone, and once again work the
color in from the roots to the ends. Be sure to work slowly
and in clean sections to keep the dye from transferring to
other zones. When finished, saran wrap if desired.

5 Zone 3 is the one farthest back, centered around the crown
of your head. It should be the easiest to apply, as the rest
of your hair is dyed at this point, so it will move around less.
Take your hair in horizontal sections and paint the color on,
again going from roots to ends.

PROCESSING

Let process at room temperature for 30 minutes and rinse with
cold water.

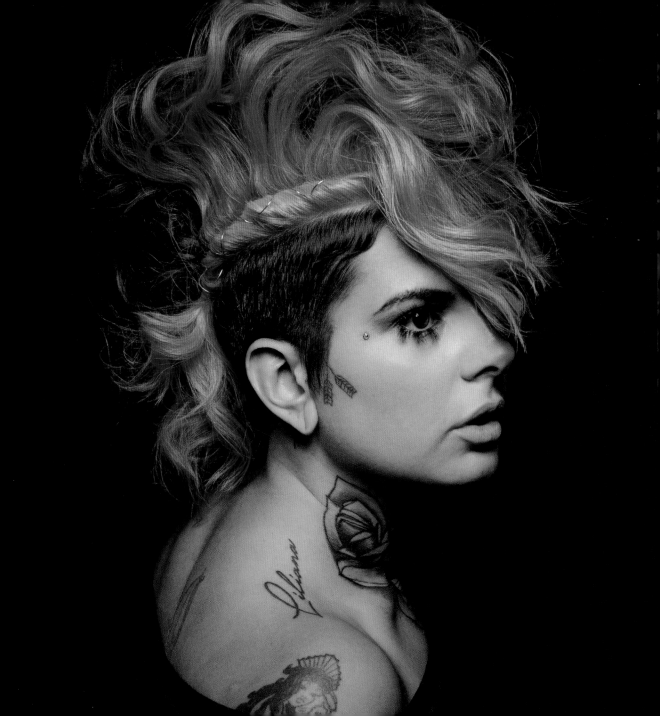

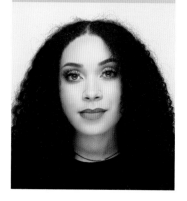

Amber's natural hair is a Level 4/5 (see the color chart on page 18).

Pro Tip

This effect is perfect for anyone who already has a balayage done and wants to spice things up! The same principles could also easily be applied to a sombre or an ombre for a different and more high-contrast look.

BALAYAGE WITH A CREATIVE COLOR OVERLAY

RASPBERRY JAM

This is a great technique for any who wants to created a graduated, natural-looking effect in fun, subtly unnatural colors.

And the best part? It's nice and easy. Just paint freehand onto the hair. Go ham!

PREPARING THE CANVAS

For this look, the first thing we did was apply a balayage to Amber's hair. Balayage is a freehand hair-painting technique, and one that we knew would be the most effective way to create dimensions using highlights, while leaving her natural hair color in some areas to become the lowlights. Her natural hair color was Level 4/5, and those darker, natural lowlights worked wonderfully, really showcasing our creative color overlay, which turned her canvas into a rich, deep Merlot.

We lifted the highlights in the balayage to a Level 8 in order to give our creative overlay a nice pop. Semipermanent color only truly anchors and adheres to hair that has been lightened, but it can still change the shade of or add some tone to the hair around it, which creates a lovely and more seamless look.

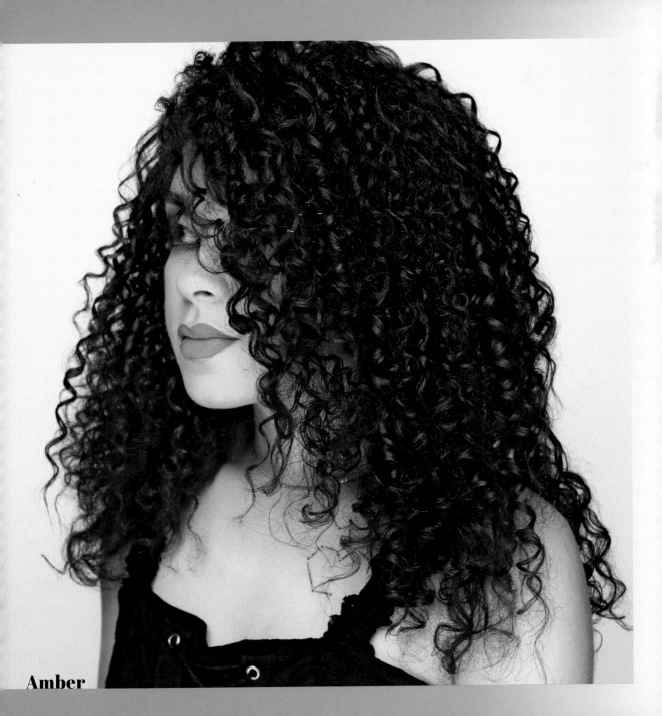

Amber

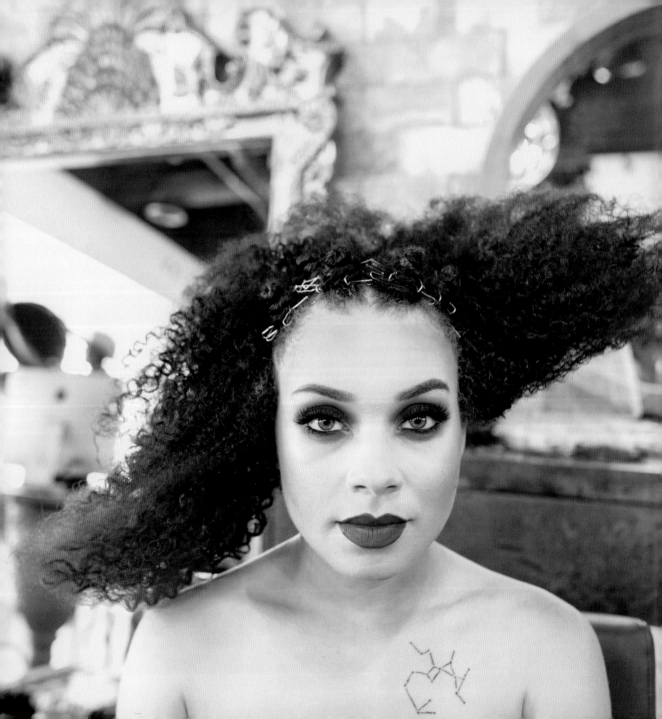

COLOR FORMULA
Overlay Formula
2 parts Bold Red + 2 parts
Deep Red + 1 part Deep Purple

APPLYING THE COLOR

1 Take a horizontal section of the hair and apply the color formula to the whole section at once, starting at the roots, then going down to the midshaft and ends.

2 Apply the color to the rest of the hair in horizontal sections, moving all the way around your head.

3 Be sure to saturate the lightened parts as fully as possible in order to get the full impact of the beautiful highlights that this technique creates.

4 Make sure there are no remaining light spots. Because this dye formulation will only fully anchor to the hair that has been lightened, you can feel free to run your fingers or a comb through your hair to spread out the dye and make sure it's thoroughly distributed.

PROCESSING
Let process at room temperature for 30 minutes and rinse with cool water until the water runs clear.

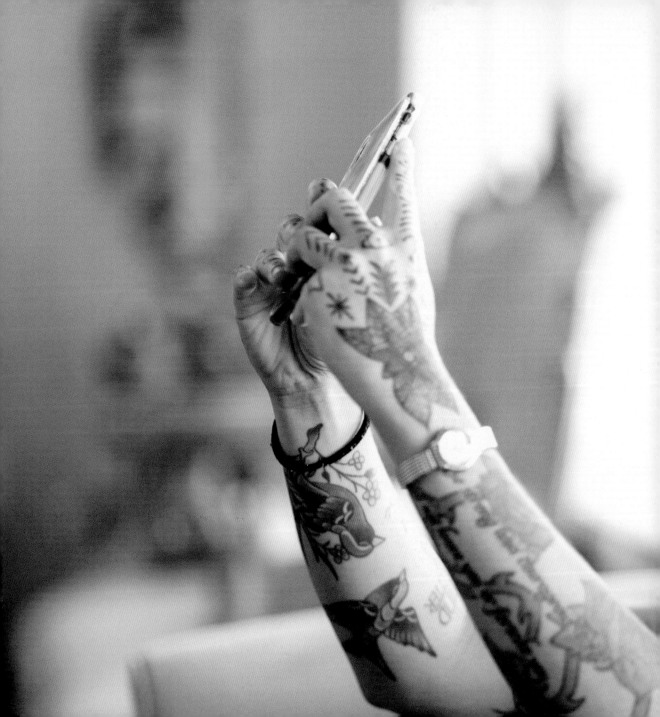

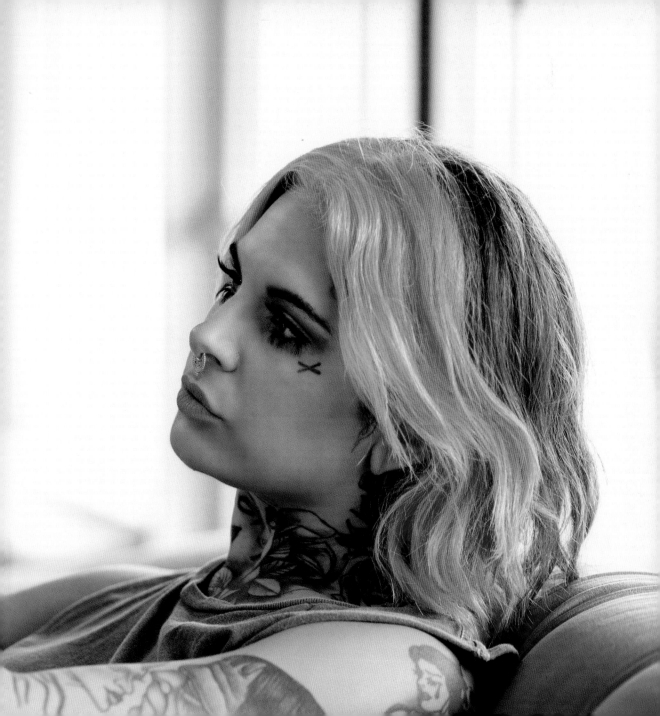

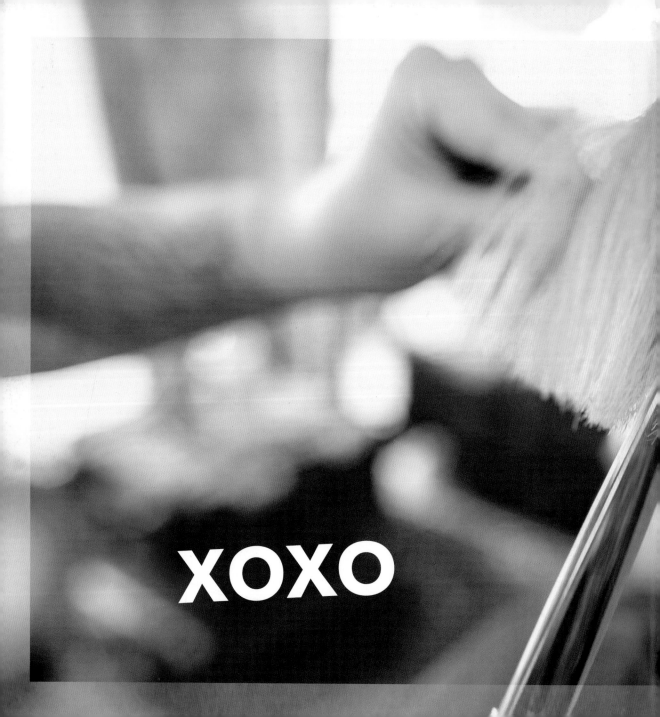

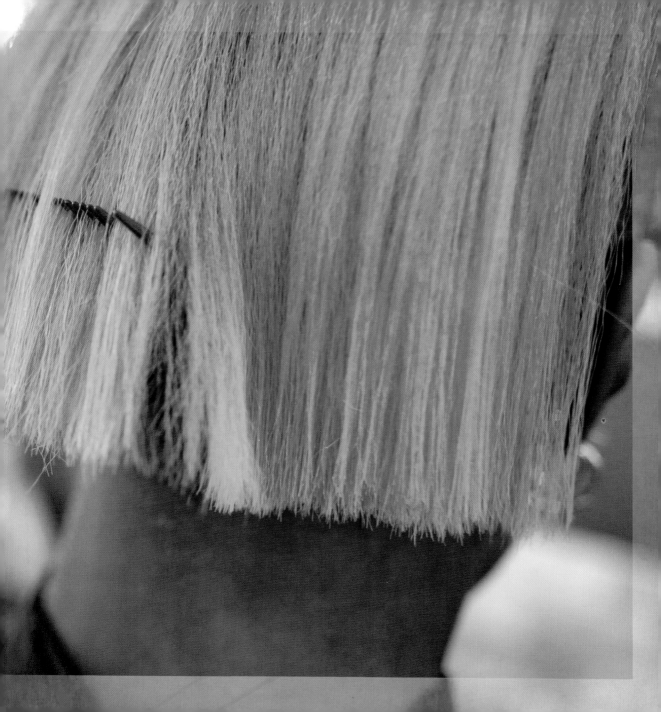

GLOSSARY

CANVAS The term that hairstylists use to refer to someone's preexisting (or recently lightened) hair—the canvas on which we put our paint (hair dye).

COLOR MELTING A technique for making sure colors transition smoothly into one another. Color melting is done by blending the edges of two different colors into each other so that they form a subtle gradient.

COLOR CORRECTING Applying one color to another (usually a contrasting color) in order to make the final color more neutral or remove an undesirable undertone. Most often, violet dye is used to color correct for the yellow and brass in bleached hair.

CROWN The very back of the top of the head, from where the hair circles outward.

DEMIPERMANENT Hair dye halfway between permanent and semipermanent in harshness and in length of effectiveness. Demipermanent hair dyes are ammonia-free, but still use a developer.

ENCAPSULATE When hair dye is left on for a long enough time (between twenty minutes and an hour, depending on the brand), it encapsulates, meaning it forms a hard shell. This hard shell is very useful, because it won't generally stain things that it touches.

ENDS The bottom of the hair. Depending on the context in which it's used, applying dye to the ends can mean either applying it to the last few inches of hair (the more traditional definition), or applying the color that extends the farthest down the hair.

FORMULA The mixture of dyes (and, in some cases, a white conditioner used to make dye lighter and create pastels) used to create the final color that will be applied to the hair.

FREEHAND PAINTING Painting dye onto the hair using a brush but without using sectioning—or, sometimes, without guidelines.

LEVEL The measurement of how light or dark a person's hair is. Note that this refers only to hair on the spectrum of possible natural colors. See the color chart on page 18 of this book for a more detailed explanation.

LIFT To lighten hair, usually by using bleach. It can refer to lightening someone's natural hair color, or to removing previously applied hair dye.

MECHE Meche strips are a very useful tool in professional hairstyling. They're clear, thin, plastic strips that are used to keep different colors of dye isolated from each other. The main benefit is that, unlike foil, they're see-through.

MIDSHAFT The middle section of a strand (or stands) of hair. The word midshaft refers to all of the hair between the roots and the ends.

NAPE The very base of the neck, where the hairline starts.

OVERLAY FORMULA A color formula applied on top of a balayage, ombre, or other technique that selectively prelightens hair. Since semi-permanent hair dyes primarily stick to lightened hair, overlay formulas can be applied over the whole head, not just the lightened portions.

PROCESS Allowing the dye to sit once applied, and be gradually absorbed into the hair. Using heat (such as a blow-dryer) will make hair dye process more quickly.

ROOTS The beginning of the hair, where the strands emerge from the head. Typically, this refers to the first two to three inches of the hair.

SECTIONING Dividing the hair into different portions, or sections, in order to make it easier to dye and ensure the dye is applied everywhere. See the Sectioning illustrations on page 24 for more details.

BRICKLAY A type of sectioning wherein hair is split into rows of blocks that are offset from each other, as in a brick wall.

DIAGONAL A type of sectioning where long, diagonal slices of hair are isolated one at a time.

HORIZONTAL The most common type of sectioning in this book, involving taking portions of hair in stripes that runs horizontally across the head.

PINWHEEL In pinwheel sectioning, all of the sections start at the crown of the head, and radiate outward.

QUADRANT The hair is divided into four different portions, or quadrants, for dye application.

VERTICAL Separating out thin, vertical strips of hair before applying dye.

SEMIPERMANENT The most common type of dye used for unnatural hair colors. Semipermanent dye is ammonia-free and conditioner-based, so it does absolutely no harm to your hair, but it doesn't last as long as the other types.

TONER Toner is a type of demipermanent color used to change the tone of the hair, usually to remove undesired yellows from bleached hair. Homemade toner can be created by mixing a bit of violet dye with white conditioner.

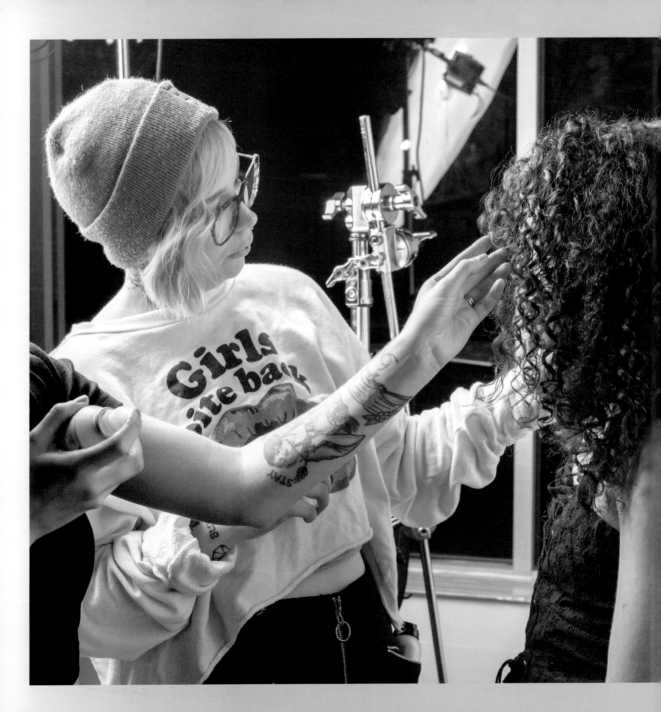

ABOUT THE AUTHOR

Ash Fortis's passion for the beauty community and dedication to education has helped her to empower hair stylists to create signature styles. Ash models her work around three core principles: Inspiration, Motivation, and Education. Her work as a stylist and in the beauty industry have been recognized by *Allure*, *The Today Show*, *BuzzFeed*, *Modern Salon*, and *American Salon*. She has also been nominated for the American Influencer Awards. Ash was a member of the original creative team that helped formulate and launch Pulp Riot. She continues to play a key role in the company, traveling and diving deeper into her passion for hair—and more importantly, the people she serves with her craft.

ACKNOWLEDGMENTS

I want to thank everyone who contributed to this book. It's been an experience I'll never forget, getting to work alongside so many beautifully talented artists. From our models, who were our greatest muses; to the makeup artists and hair stylists who brought everything together with their creative visions; to our photography team, who captured each shot so wonderfully. I especially want to thank my family and the XO Hair Lab team for their incredible support throughout the making of this book: I couldn't have done this without you, or without the incredible Weldon Owen team.

HAIR STYLISTS

Jodi Kurpiel, Rebecca Wylie, Megan Bailey, Alec Cynova, Erin Wilson, Kaitlyn Hackforth, Gianna Lidgett, Dee Marie, Michael Bargallo, Nathan Flippo, Mandi Brooks, Catherine Gibbs, Jacob Lee

MAKEUP AND MAKEUP ARTISTS

Lead makeup artist: Rebecca Whylie. Anna Oliynyk, Rachel Martino, Gaby Roby, Empress Simons, Karyn Brogan, Kaitlyn Lounsberry

Special thanks to Sarah Rillion and her amazing makeup artists, from The Makeup School by Sarah Rillion.

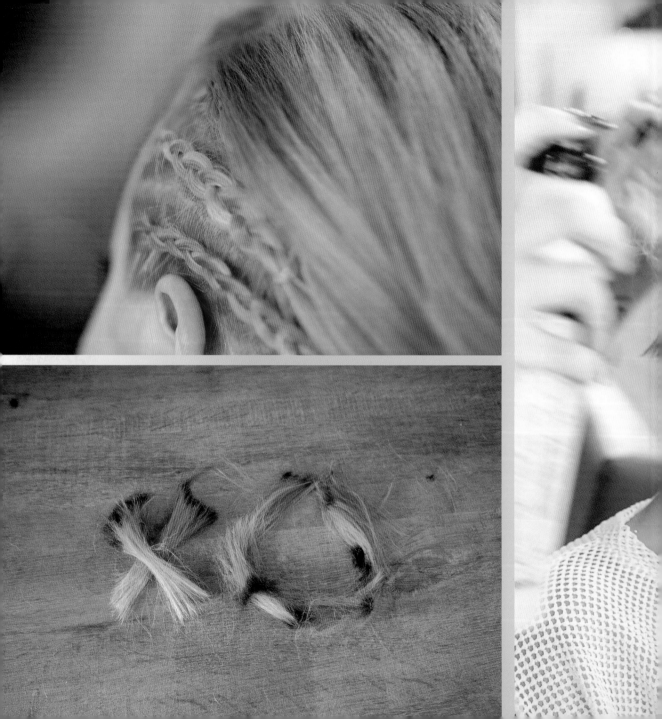

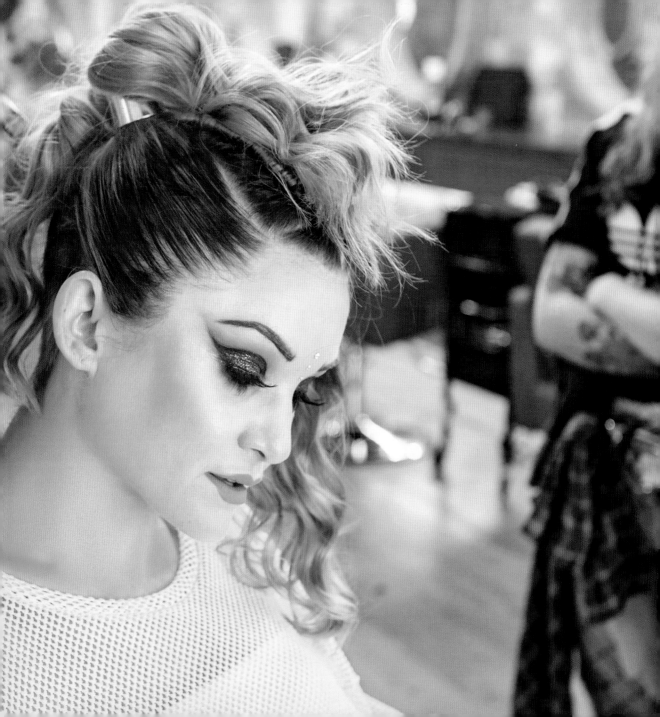

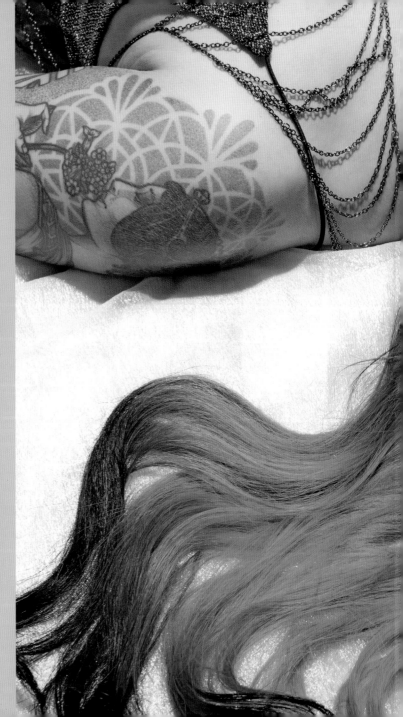

weldon**owen**

CEO Raoul Goff

President Kate Jerome

Publisher Roger Shaw

Associate Publisher Mariah Bear

Creative Director Chrissy Kwasnik

Art Director Allister Fein

Designer and Photo Art Director
Angela Williams

Editor Ian Cannon

Editorial Assistant Madeleine Calvi

Managing Editor Tarji Rodriguez

Production Manager Binh Au

Weldon Owen would like to thank
Jessica Lack for copyediting. All photos
by Glenn Fajota with the exception of
images by Ben Hoedt (pages 14–15 and
22–23) and those provided by Pulp Riot
(pages 18–21). Conor Buckley of And
Them created illustrations.

1150 Brickyard Cove Road
Richmond, CA 94801
www.weldonowen.com

ISBN 13: 978-1-68188-504-9

10 9 8 7 6 5 4 3 2 1
2020 2021 2022 2023

Printed in China

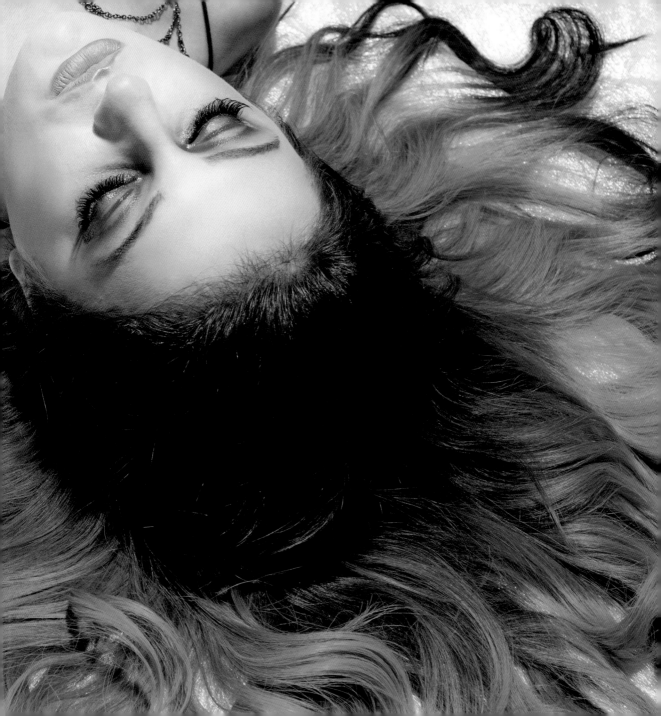

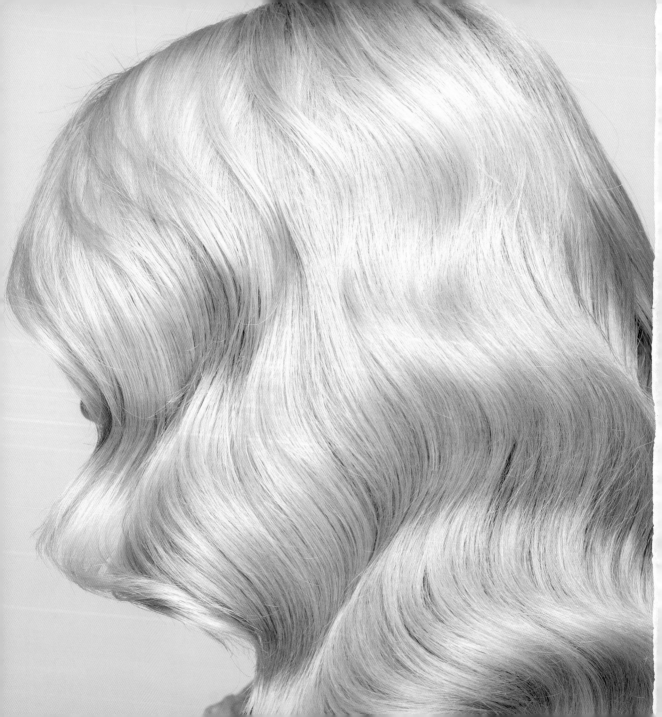